THE SNEAKY AF* DIET BOOK

THE SNEAKY AF* DIET BOOK

LOSE WEIGHT AND FEEL GREAT WITHOUT EVEN TRYING

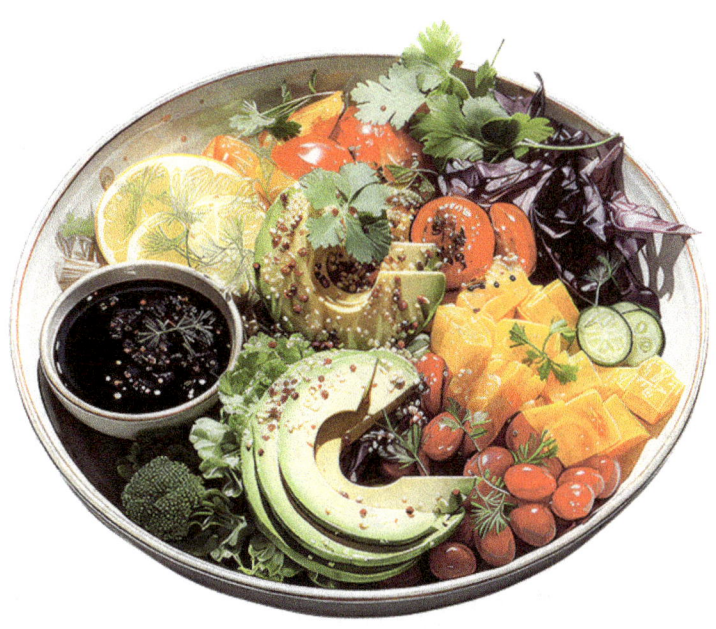

©COPYWRITE 2024 – ALL RIGHTS RESERVED

Feel Good Publishing

Los Angeles, California

Copyright © 2024 by Feel Good Publishing

All rights reserved.

No portion of this book may be reproduced in any form without written permission from the author and/or publisher, except as permitted by U.S. copyright law.

This publication is designed to provide accurate and authoritative information about nutrition and wellness. It is sold with the understanding that neither the author nor the publisher guarantees the information as statistically complete as new studies may render some information incomplete.

While the publisher and author have used their best efforts in preparing this book, they make no representations or warranties concerning the accuracy or completeness of the contents of this book that you are guaranteed to lose weight. This book is a guideline to living a healthier life.

The author and/or publisher specifically disclaim any implied warranties of fitness and wellness. The advice and strategies contained herein may not be suitable for your situation. You should consult with a professional or physician when appropriate. Neither the publisher nor the author shall be liable for any loss, including but not limited to special, incidental, consequential, personal, or other damages.

About the Author

Sarah Rutherford was born and raised in Melbourne, Australia. She was an avid horse rider and loved spending summers at the beach.

She moved to California in 1996. She has spent much time exploring food and culture in Europe and South America.

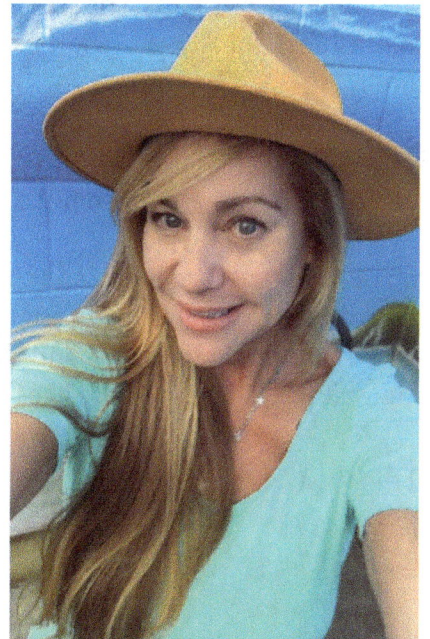

She has always had a fascination nutrition with and wellness.

She studied her 200-hour Yoga Teacher Training in Koh Phangan, Thailand. Five years later she completed her additional 300 hours YTT in India.

This has taken her on a journey of wellness, alternative medicine, and nutrition.

Sarah has always seen a direct correlation between food and wellness. She is a keen cook and enjoys showing friends and family just how delicious a plant-based menu can taste.

She is a keen believer in approaching plant medicines to cure ailments in instances where they can be equally effective as pharmaceuticals.

Sarah ran a CBD (non-psychoactive cannabinoid) manufacturing and retail business for 4 years and has seen firsthand the ability to heal naturally.

This book is a culmination of 3 years of research and a lifetime of trial and error with eating nourishing foods and diets.

Sarah believes balance is key and she believes you can have your cake and eat it too... literally.
We hope you enjoy this book and that it helps you to make profound changes in your life and in the lives of your loved ones.

Bon Appetit!

Preamble

You cannot offend an animal because they speak a different language.

"Every act of animal abuse diminishes our collective humanity. We must work together to create a world free from cruelty and violence."
— *Sangdeun Chailert*

"We must remember that our actions towards animals reflect our humanity. It is our responsibility to be compassionate and kind."
— *Velma Bronn Johnston*

Table of Contents

Chapter 1 *How did food get so confusing?* 1

Chapter 2 *So how does Food Combining (Trophology) fit into the Equation?* 13

Chapter 3 *Choose Organic* 21

Chapter 4 *Does mTOR Help or Hinder?* 25

Chapter 5 *High Protein Diets – The Myth* 31

Chapter 6 *Water Consumption* 37

Chapter 7 *Is Sugar Good or Bad for my health?* 41

Chapter 8 *Gut Health & Improving Your Microbiome* 43

Chapter 9 *You Can Help the Environment* 49

Chapter 10 *The Scientific Evidence Is Overwhelming* 53

Chapter 11 *Become a Flexitarian!* 63

Chapter 12 *Blue Zones* 67

Chapter 13 *Diet vs Hereditary* 89

Chapter 14 *But Animals are Tasty* 95

Chapter 15 *Choose Alternatives* 101

Chapter 16 *Isn't Eating Plant Based Expensive?* 109

Chapter 17 *Fasting/Cleanses* 113

Chapter 18 *The 8 Limbs of Yoga* 119

Chapter 19 *The Chakras* 137

Chapter 20 *Laughter is the best Medicine!* 147

Chapter 21 *The Gratitude Jar* 151

Chapter 22 *Meditation* 155

Chapter 23 *How to Increase Neurotransmitters Naturally* .. 159

Chapter 24 *Enduro India - The Adventure of a Lifetime* 177

Chapter 25 *A Plant-based Week* 183

Chapter 26 *Be Part of the Plant-based Revolution!* 193

Glossary of Plant Medicines 201

Preface

I strongly believe I was born a vegan. I like to believe that I was a Buddhist monk in my last life, and I decided I'd like to come by as a hot-ish carefree little Australian, free as a bird.

I distinctly remember my mother packing my school lunches. The sandwich always contained meat and often cheese. Each day I would throw them in the trash. I hated meat as a child. Growing up in the 1970s in Australia, my Mum believed that the 3 of us kids needed meat and vegetables.

I was pale and skinny. I was definitely unhealthy-looking. I remember my uncle securing my sister and I a pictorial advertising campaign. We needed to stand there and look pretty, as I recall we needed to pretend to be someone's nieces for a print media campaign. We were paid $90 each but they couldn't use the photos because I looked so sickly and pale.

I became so skinny at one point that Mum took me to the doctor. By today's standards, I would have been labeled anorexic. Thankfully back then this was not an option. It may well have changed the trajectory of my life in a negative way. Who likes labels? *(Unless they are on a designer bag or coat... of course.)*

Also, (not thankfully) – ADHD was not a diagnosis back then. It would have helped me no end if I had been prescribed the necessary medication back in the 1970's so I could actually concentrate on one thing.

The doctor told my mother to feed me whatever I felt like eating.

So, each day for several months – I ate nothing but pancakes. She'd still make the meat and vegetables for dinner, and I'd pick at the meal without consuming much, except for the vegetables.

Then I went through a toasted banana sandwich stage. That single one phase may have lasted around 5-6 months. Kudos to my Mum for tolerating my requests for somewhat vegan foods. I probably drove her nuts. I gained weight from age 8 years old – 12 years old. Her desire to feed me whichever food I would eat, and not force me to eat specific foods, probably helped me to flourish.

When we are in tune with them, I strongly believe our bodies tell us what we need and require for nourishment. It is developing this necessary harmonious relationship with our inner selves that will lead us to a place of happiness.

Listen. Your body will talk to you. I promise.

Chapter 1
How did food get so confusing?

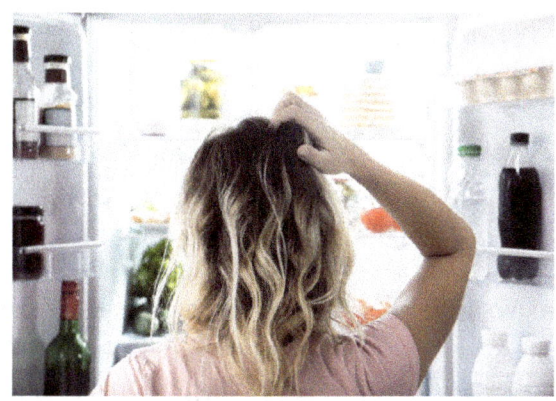

We all just want to be healthy, right? We want to live full lives. We want our kids to grow up and be strong. We want our parents to grow old and grumpy *(joke)* surrounded by grandkids. That's what we want. Community, purpose, harmony. How did choosing a healthy diet become so difficult?

Supermarkets are packed full of pre-made foods claiming to be healthy but how do we ultimately get through all the BS and eat what we should be eating? Without breaking the bank? And of course, without taking up our precious free time.

THE SNEAKY AF* DIET BOOK

We all ultimately want the same things in life. To live to a grand old age surrounded by people who love us, and that we love unconditionally.

The destination is amazing. We have the backpack. We brought our snacks. We even brought sunscreen……. but somehow the road seems to crumble beneath our feet. And if we are fortunate enough to make it to our 80th birthday without getting hit by illness or disease then we are the lucky ones. I like to look at life as if I'm a builder laying down bricks one in front of the other. Paving his or her own road. These building blocks are diet, exercise, and purpose. They all lead us to a wonderful destination.

I am no Saint. I have done my fair share of partying in my younger years. It has taken me a lifetime of research to share what I have learned with you. Mistakes and all. I have made many of those!

At the time of writing this book, I have turned 50 years of age. And I would like to be here for another 50 years. And this has prompted me to research longevity, and more specifically – diet. It's important to change the road now. Me especially. More specifically to make up for the years of excess and enjoyment.

Choosing a healthy path need not necessarily dictate deprivation. In fact, the complete opposite is achievable. I promise! We all need to pave the way to a healthy and happy future, especially if we want to live to a grand old age. Not just for ourselves, but also for our families and loved ones. And not to mention, we also have due diligence to preserve our wonderful planet. She provides us with a bounty and diversity so rich.

So, how did our diets and our lifestyles get so messed up?

There is no single answer. It could partly be due to busy schedules. We have all felt like this. Overstretched in our commitments to family and work with barely much time to devote to our wellbeing. Convenience plays a big factor here. It is little surprising that fast food chains, which often result in unhealthy choices, have become prolific in the Western world.

As our lives get more and more hectic, it is often preferable to find a fast-food shortcut to save precious time in order to get through the day. The fast-food industry was birthed out of this very concept. Time is a precious commodity that we can never get back. However, eating a predominantly plant-based diet does not have to be difficult. And it doesn't have to be all-or-nothing.

A healthy balance can be achieved. And this most certainly can be different for every individual.

We need to pave that road every day with the right building blocks to pave the way to a happier and healthier future. And I am not saying give up meat and dairy altogether. It's more about making healthy smart choices and limiting the amount of cholesterol we consume from animal products.

The only contributor to cholesterol levels and heart disease is the animal fat derived from meat and dairy clogging our arteries and bloodstream. Heart disease is the number one killer in the world.

We are bombarded with information and nutritional facts. This particular celebrity did a juice cleanse and lost 20 lbs, this athlete only eats protein and no carbohydrates. It has become so confusing that it is hard to know what is healthy and what is not.

THE SNEAKY AF* DIET BOOK

We have become hyper-focused on fad diets instead of becoming acutely aware of the foods we are combining. We will delve into this in delve a little later. *(Chapter on Trophology)*

We have many of the 'so-called health gurus' saying don't eat this, but you can eat that. Eating avocados is one of my favorite examples, long vilified for being high in fat, it seems now most experts can agree they are rich in 'good fat'. More about that later. Counting calories, lowering carbohydrates, restricting portion control, eating more vegetables, eating less sugar, intermittent fasting… the list goes on and on.

But what if I told you there was an easier way? A simpler way. To lose weight. To feel great. To get your health back. To take control of not just your future but also your destiny. You'd think there is a catch, right? No catch.

Just add in a few days a week when you will eat entirely plant-based foods. Up your water intake. Take a couple of enjoyable short strolls after meals (or any exercise you like). And before you know it you will have lost weight.

Plant-based foods can be amazingly tasty and guess what? It's sustainable. When I throw around words like sustainability it is not just to appear empathetic and planet conscious.

We have surpassed a planet with 8 billion humans living on it. And the current model of dairy farming and meat production cannot sustain feeding this population without some extremely dire consequences.

In a few decades, this book will probably become obsolete because some smarty pants scientist will have worked a way to grow meat in a lab. Even if that does happen, I think I'll stick with my current 80% plant-based diet/20% whatever *the fuck* I want to eat. Over the last year, I have lost almost 15 pounds. I sleep better and I feel great! Not bad for a 50-year-old who still likes a few more than the occasional cocktail and is allergic to the gym. To my credit, I do yoga *almost* every day.

I can sense many of you yawning right now thinking this is another preachy vegan book. Hell to no! Having tried going vegan in my 20's (the year is 1998!) I made it to about the 6-month mark and I quit unexpectedly one night.

I was leaving for a 6-week vacation in Thailand, Cambodia & Laos and one of my friends suggested I stay the night at her house before departing. Unbeknownst to me, she had organized a surprise birthday party as I was going to be in Thailand on my actual birthday and she believed in celebrating a birthday 'month' not just a day.

My boyfriend and I arrived, and we were delighted to see balloons tied around each individual chair at the dining table. I didn't put two and two together, so I asked, 'Whose party is this?'. My friend replied 'Well, yours of course!'. I must have subconsciously noted the aromas of lamb baking in the oven as I was beginning to salivate.

Lamb is one of my absolute, all-time favorite things to eat. Having grown up in Australia, we are a nation of lamb devourers. In every form… kababs, shawarmas, your sophisticated rack of lamb, and of course the good old fashioned Sunday roast leg of lamb, which was what my friend had baked in the oven for my birthday dinner.

THE SNEAKY AF* DIET BOOK

We had a fabulous evening. She had invited many of our mutual friends. The food was delicious. I didn't even question breaking my 6-month vegan lifestyle for one second. Perhaps it was the 5th glass of red wine. Or the promise of my departing flight the following day to faraway lands and mystical travels. On that night I slipped back into my old meat-eating ways like I had just gone to bed last night with pork chop grease on my lips.

What surprised me upon arrival in Thailand, is that they are predominantly meat eaters. Like serious, *chicken hanging from a string with its feather on*, in the market, meat eaters. But they were all relatively slim. There were a few fatties but not nearly as many as I was used to seeing in America. (I mean no offense by the term 'fatties' – I am an Australian, so hopefully that will make my questionable commentary exempt for the remainder of the book. And the unforeseen future).

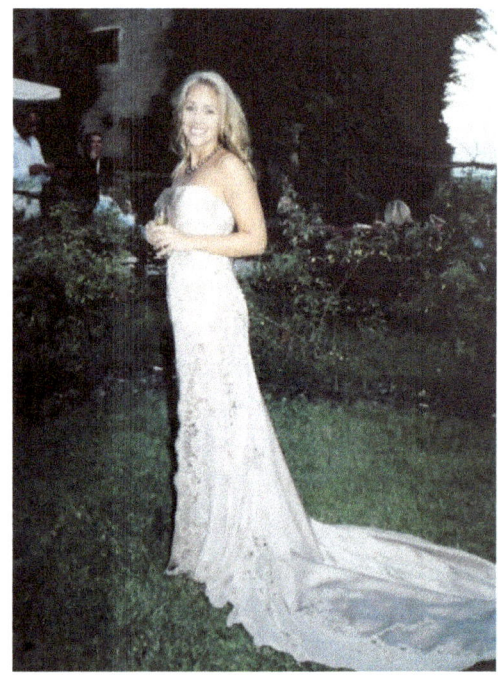

These people were slim and gorgeous. Genealogy? Perhaps. Lack of preservatives and fresh healthy food? My wager is on the latter.

I continued to eat meat. All through the 6-week vacation and on my return to Los Angeles. We were getting married. I wanted to look svelte and amazing for my wedding as does every bride-to-be.

As it drew nearer to my wedding I was working out with a trainer and eating minimal carbohydrates, protein shakes... egg whites. I was quite slim, but I definitely didn't feel good. I figured that was the price you paid for looking hot-ish. I was lethargic and suffered from brain fog. This restrictive way of eating only 1500 calories a day was not for me.

On a side note, I have always been on the spectrum of hot *(good-looking)*. Not quite hot, but almost hot. It really is more problematic than being either plain or very good-looking. I feel that now I have surpassed my 50th birthday (the year is 2022) I am going to be one of those hot old ladies. You see her and you say, she must have been gorgeous when she was young (another attempt at humor). But boy it looks like she had some fun!

Back to the part about me being previously vegan... for a whole 6 months...

When I say 'vegan' I wasn't a hard and fast vegan. I still ate vegetable dishes from our local Indian restaurant which were sure to contain ghee which is a form of clarified butter Indians use in their cooking.

It was a wonderful trip to Asia. I wasn't restricted by what I was eating. I became a carnivore again and never looked back.

I was married in Italy. In a castle. Seriously. I got married in a castle. I have photos to prove it. I say this because many people around me looked at me as if they were thinking 'How did this little Aussie get here?'.

I fit right into my teeny, tiny wedding dress and I believe I looked fabulous on the day. It took a lot of work. I wish I'd known how easy it is to go plant-based and lose weight without trying!

THE SNEAKY AF* DIET BOOK

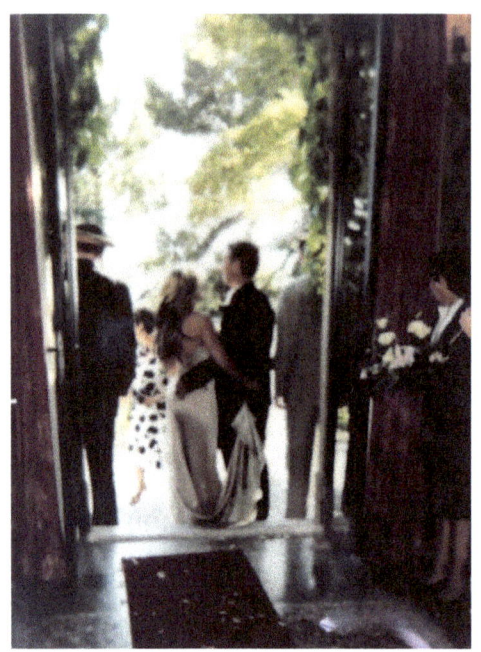

This diet of meat eating, and no carbohydrates seemed to suit me well from the outside, but I often felt a bit sick and definitely not satiated. However, I was quite slim. I felt deprived. I was a bit sad honestly.

I think it was around 18 months later that I moved to England. I had always been a healthy eater in California. The weather is warm, so I ate a lot of salads and light faire along with meat and dairy.

England is cold most of the year. It's dreary and dull in winter. There is not a lot to do except go to the pub and eat. England is a wonderful place to vacation for the six weeks of summer. The rest of the time it's pretty bleak, to be honest. I highly recommend you research when these 6 weeks of summer will occur if you plan on visiting. If you do not hear the irony in my tone – you have clearly never been to England.

The weather is conducive to eating meat-based, heavy dishes. Stews and curries, roast beef with Yorkshire puddings, roast potatoes with lashings of lard-based gravy.

I remembered an early trip to England with my lamb roast birthday dinner pal. We had a rather interesting flight.

We were just two-party gals off on another adventure. *(This is pre-vegan phase.)* I believe this was the Atkins diet phase because I do remember having about 20 Atkins bars in my luggage.

No one had ever mentioned to us that sleeping tablets should probably not be consumed with alcohol. Upon boarding our flight and being upgraded to business class we said yes to the complimentary champagne. Yes, to all the food and drinks. And we decided we should get some rest – so why not take an Ambien?

We awoke in a fuzzy haze. I remember looking at my friend and wondering why she had white panda eyes. Oh, that would be due to the $290 eye cream we had bought along with an aged bottle of scotch duty-free in our wine/pill-induced shopping spree on the plane.

We had arrived at London Heathrow, and we were hungry and hangry too, *(oh and hungover)*!

Our friend Robin picked us up from the airport. He, in his wisdom, recognized our 'hanger' (hungry + impending anger) and decided that a truck stop brekkie would hit the spot. He said it was the best place for 'The Full English Breakfast'. A notorious English delicacy containing greasy sausages, bacon, eggs, beans, tomatoes, black pudding, and toast. I asked the waitress for my toast 'with no butter'. She replied, rather snappily, 'It's fried'. Yes, the bread was deep-fried! How novel. Talk about an artery blocker.

We had a fabulous vacation. I was still a bit overweight. I never really understood what to eat or in which order. I wish someone had explained it to me back then. *But if they did, I most certainly wouldn't be writing this book!*

It was not until I moved to England in 2003 that my somewhat healthy food choices went out the window pretty much.

My time spent in England opened me up to fabulous meat-based, and cream-based sauce dishes. Potatoes fried in duck fat. Pies. The kind with meat in the middle. Clotted cream. And all the while I was adding 5lbs to my petite frame each year which does not sound like a lot but over 6 years it can really add up.

I remember my Mum coming to visit me in England. She'd flown out from Australia. I was a bit overweight. I remember she commented on how just gaining 5lbs a year, can really add up over a 6-year time span.

Determined to take control of my health I booked in to do an intensive one-month yoga teacher training in Thailand. I'd always loved yoga, but I was hardly in shape! I just knew something had to change.

My most favorite part of this story is that whilst my drinking has remained somewhat in control over the past few years, it does have the propensity to get out of hand. I figured completing a yoga teacher training was cheaper than rehab. Think about it.. $3,000 for Yoga Teacher Training vs $30,000 for rehab. Been to both. My money is on the yoga teacher training. *Just some free advice.* Yoga works way better, and it is way much fun. *(More about the 8 limbs of yoga later – if I can hold your attention for that long).*

It was precisely what I needed. One month away with no alcohol and eating only healthy foods. Just yoga, the beach, and good times. I know Thailand. I have been to Thailand. I can do this.

No husband.

Definitely a plus.

I immersed myself in the culture. It was mind-expanding. I was diligent and took notes. Our yoga teacher was absolutely amazing, and I was gaining back my inner strength. My mental clarity was acute, and I felt the best I had felt in a very long time. I could do this. I remember thinking 'I am going to be thin and hot-ish again'.

I was on Koh Phangan and I think there were drugs on the island. In fact, I knew there were drugs on the island.

Our yoga teacher's rule was no drugs and no drinking, so we diligently showed up to each class. We learned. We shone.

One of the students on the course introduced me to a way of eating called combining specific foods, at specific times of the day, based on the scientific principle of Trophology. And Trophology served me well. All through my 30's and early 40's, I was able to stay slim and eat pretty much what I wanted. The only restriction was eating certain foods at certain times of the day. The science of Food Combining is a great practice if you want to continue to eat meat and dairy and I will base a chapter on this next.

I will never truly know if it was the food combining or the party scene, which kept me slim throughout my 30's and 40's. I do know one thing. I had a lot of fun, and I wouldn't trade those memories for all the gold in the world.

But as I entered my late forties it just stopped working and I am left wondering why. Maybe I got lazy and bent the rules a bit. Maybe I was more settled, but I had to leave the partying phase of my life behind. It doesn't serve one well into their 40's and 50's.

So, I decided to set about learning as much about nutrition and plant medicine as possible. This book is a culmination of that knowledge.

Chapter 2
So how does Food Combining (Trophology) fit into the Equation?

Trophology is the science of food combining. It is not a new concept. In fact, it has been around for thousands of years. It has been bandied around over the past 5 or 6 decades often rolled out as a new diet such as the Hay Diet, Food Combining, Evolved Eating, etc.

Tropology is highly effective, as it is a scientific principle, which works on the simple basic premise of gut digestion and pH balance.

When we masticate (chew) our food, our body senses the chemical breakdown of the food, based on the reactive saliva which sends signals to the brain. The brain then signals to our stomach to release digestive enzymes to break down the food, so that it may pass through the digestive tract effectively and efficiently.

Carbohydrates require an alkaline digestive environment. The saliva signals our brain to release the digestive enzyme *ptyalin* into our digestive tract. Meat and dairy require an acidic digestive environment. This digestive enzyme is called *pepsin*.

So, what happens when we eat a burger with fries and throw in a sugary milkshake to boot? Complete chaos in the digestive tract!

The body releases both acidic enzymes and alkaline enzymes. The carbohydrates require ptyalin and the meat and dairy require pepsin. And when they all arrive at the party in the stomach, they end up neutralizing each other and becoming completely inefficient. Thus, this kind of meal cannot be effectively digested which is why we often feel bloated or lethargic after eating such a feast.

Our food sits in a water-like environment with no ability to digest. This is often why a big meal, like the one mentioned above, leaves us feeling bloated, tired, and entirely not well.

It all comes down to the pH scale, which exists in our digestive tract. Think about a swimming pool. What do we do if the water is too acidic? We make it more alkaline. And if it's too alkaline we make it more acidic. We want a neutral pH.

We want a neutral water environment in our swimming pool, but we definitely do not want this environment in our guts if we are to digest food efficiently and effectively.

A meal of a lettuce-wrapped burger and an unsweetened iced tea would be far easier to digest as our body would release acidic enzymes called pepsin. It would have none of the sugars or very few carbohydrates to contend with and it would be able to process this food comparatively quickly compared to the standard burger, fries, and milkshake.

If you love a burger, fries and a milkshake – I challenge you to ask for the burger with a veggie patty (if they do not offer this simply ask for it with no meat and cheese) and sub the milkshake for an unsweetened iced tea. Sometimes, I will add some French fries to my burger (no meat) and get the burger patty on the side for my dog. No salt or seasoning of course. Dogs are carnivores. They were designed to be. However, we are not.

Guage how you feel after eating this meal vs eating your regular burger, french fries, and milkshake.

Now I do not advocate doing this all the time. I will occasionally do this when I am on a road trip, and I am short on time. I still eat junk food occasionally. I actually enjoy it. But again, everything in moderation. If we start to adopt an 80/20 balance (80% healthy plant-based foods and 20% foods we enjoy but are not necessarily great for us) then we become more prone to make healthy decisions. But we can still eat out at our favorite restaurants or show up to a dinner party without looking like a *vegan asshole*.

Below is the food-combining pyramid according to a food-combining model. It shows you exactly which foods combine well with others, as well as food combinations to avoid.

THE SNEAKY AF* DIET BOOK

The Food Combining Pyramid

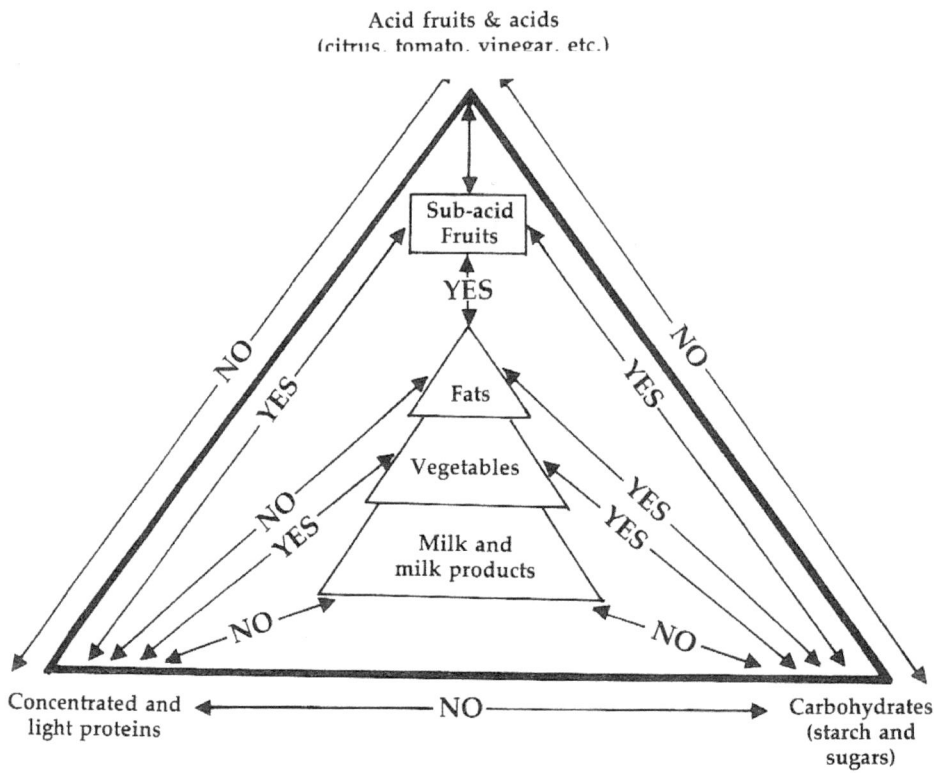

Similarly, a carbohydrate-based meal with little to no protein of a vegetable pasta with no meat and no dairy would pass quite quickly through the digestive tract as it would only require an alkaline environment (ptyalin enzyme) to digest efficiently.

Our stomachs work in the same manner. So, when we load them up with a weird combination of foods that are both carbohydrate-based and made up of animal fats and proteins, our bodies release too many counter-active digestive enzymes negating the effects of each of the individual enzymes. This leads to poor digestion. It can also lead to meat rotting in the intestines as it cannot pass through the body quickly enough and it becomes rancid. Rotting food in the intestines can lead to cancer and disease.

If you are a die-hard meat and dairy eater, then you need to change the way you consume these products if you want to live to a healthy old age. And we most certainly know we need to eat less animal protein-rich foods as we age.

Eating meat with green leafy vegetables or salads will allow them to digest more rapidly. This is because there are minimal carbohydrates in green leafy vegetables and salads.

This system of eating served me well for almost 20 years but now as I near my 50's I have found that my body cannot tolerate meat or dairy well. I also have a sensitivity to gluten, so I tend to avoid gluten-heavy foods or find handy alternatives to substitute gluten-rich foods that I enjoy occasionally like pasta or bagels.

A side word here about processed meats like cold cuts, hot dogs, salami, pepperoni, and many of the deli meats that many of us have consumed throughout our lives. These foods are carcinogenic and should be avoided. The addition of chemicals and preservatives makes them highly toxic to the body.

When choosing meat – it is always a good idea to pay the extra money for farm-raised, antibiotic-free free, and hormone-free meat, eggs, and dairy. It is more expensive but if you cut the portion size by half it will offset the price difference and you may even save a little.

I order Butcher Box every few months. It's organic grass-fed meat and seafood. I love to have steaks and meat on hand for if I am entertaining.

I am quite partial to a small filet of wild-caught salmon, cauliflower rice (low carbs), and green vegetables. I eat this once a week. It doesn't have to be all or nothing.

I have three or four days a week where I eat completely plant-based and I do not miss meat or dairy at all.

Food Combining Chart

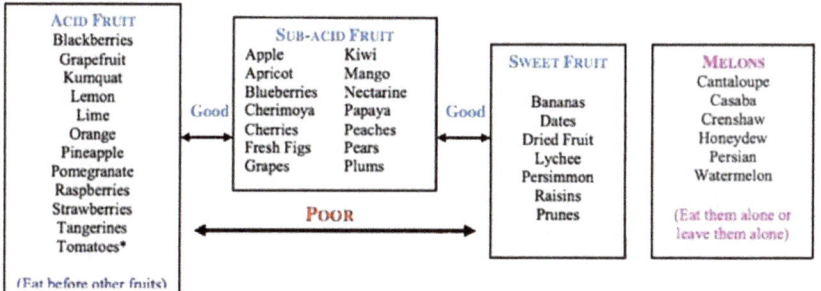
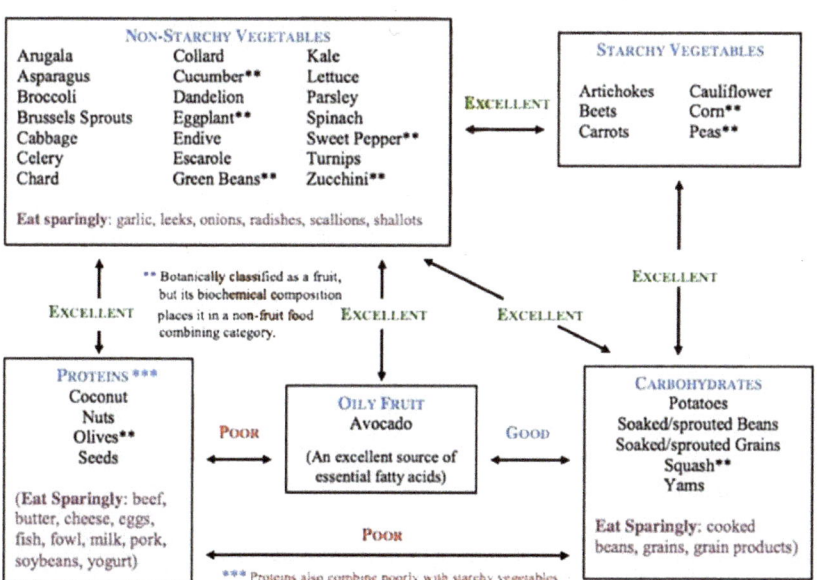

THE SNEAKY AF* DIET BOOK

Chapter 3
Choose Organic

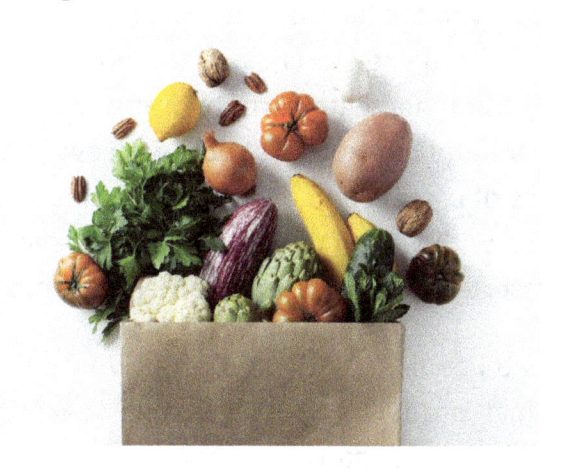

Studies show us that organically grown foods have far higher amounts of Vitamin C, iron, magnesium, phosphorus, and nitrates than fruits and vegetables grown with fertilizers and pesticides. Chemical pesticides have been linked to numerous diseases including birth defects.

Not only are fertilizers linked to a decrease in essential nutrients they are also increasing the risk of cancer.

Purchasing organic produce has a profound effect on the environment too. Wildlife thrives around crops grown organically. Frogs, insects, birds, and, wildlife can all thrive with the abstinence of damaging pesticides and poison.

Pesticides make their way into the water table polluting not just the immediate area, but also the land for thousands of miles around.

It is important to note that plant-based proteins don't necessarily apply to the laws of Trophology. Why? Because plant proteins are treated like starches by the body. This means they can be easily combined with carbohydrates. Eat lentils and rice. Eat mung beans and potatoes. Eat nuts with everything! They are a great source of protein and an amazing replacement for cream when blended with water. Cashew cream is delicious. It can be added to desserts or can be used as a delicious pasta sauce.

Once I realized I could make one of my favorite things on earth without animal products I realized that vegan can be more delicious and healthier than any other meal.

I love carbonara pasta. I've made it since I was in my 20's. There are times in my life when have only eaten it occasionally because whatever diet or eating regime I was on, occluded it from my dietary repertoire. But I'd still eat it occasionally.

Once I found I could blend ½ cup raw cashews and ½ cup of water to make cream and that I could buy delicious plant-based 'benevolent bacon' I realized I could eat this dish every week and never gain weight.

In fact, now when I do eat the wrong foods (and it's easy to do with a hectic lifestyle) I find my body feeling sluggish, and I find myself sleeping more. I start to crave healthy plant-based alternatives.

I found if I could substitute many of my go-to lunch foods with plant-based ingredients life would be smooth sailing. I routinely have several tubs of acai sorbet in the fridge at work and at home. I freeze bananas. I have blueberries in the fridge. I add gluten-free granola, goji berries, and some nut butter, and whammo! I have a delicious lunch or snack.

I bulk-buy raw nuts and roast them in the oven adding a tiny amount of maple syrup and some bagel seasoning and this serves as the perfect snack.

Salads can be jazzed up with the addition of seeds, nuts or cranberries. Sweet potato and quinoa are a wonderful addition.

Many supermarkets have amazing easy-to-prepare freezer meals like meatless orange chicken. Vegan curries. Plant-based green goddess bowls. And while these are not necessarily the best choice, they are perfect in a pinch. They save me from making an unhealthy choice. There is even an abundance of fast-food options. And while I DO NOT advocate eating fast food often, I get it – TIME IS OUR MOST PRECIOUS COMMODITY.

Now, I find if I make large batches of foods I enjoy and then freeze smaller portions, I can live (almost) entirely without needing to buy fast food or processed foods.

The other wonderful benefit of eating plant-based is that you will find you are less hungry and less often. I always thought I had some kind of blood sugar issue. I would get extremely hungry, and often moody if I went longer than 4 hours without food.

Now I find I can go for longer periods of time without even feeling necessarily hungry. However, I do always carry a few snacks in my car, like the roast nuts mentioned above.

Rome wasn't built in a day. I am not an advocate of all or nothing. Making changes and adjusting your diet can take time and energy but I 100% guarantee you it will be worth it in the long run.

You don't have to commit to changing your diet completely. Perhaps just commit to one full day a week eating only plant-based. If you feel better, perhaps you will add another day and another….

And before you know it you will find that eating plant-based is easy and it will keep you slim. And healthy!

There are a million more reasons to eat plant-based than just for losing weight, but if that is your motivation – then that is perfectly fine!

Chapter 4
Does mTOR Help or Hinder?

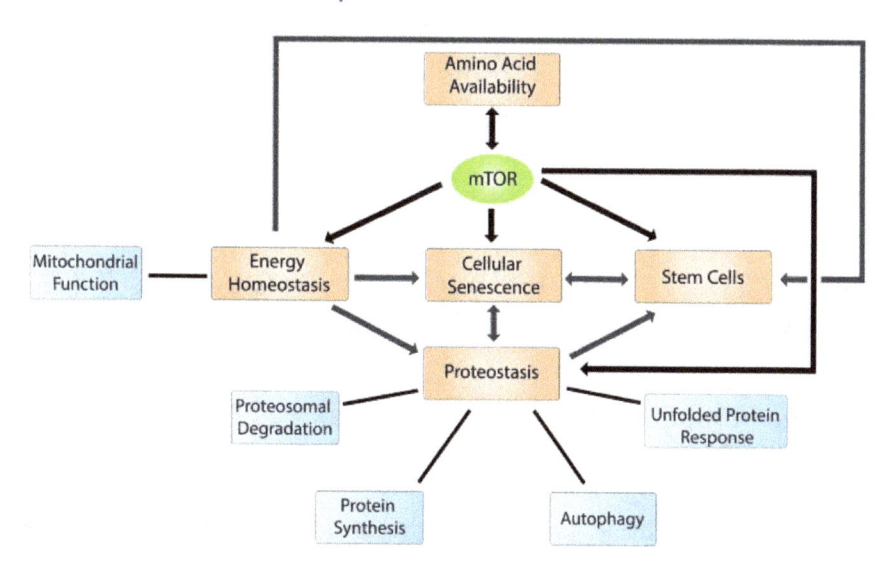

The human body has a special protein called mammalian target of rapamycin (mTOR). Research has shown that it is responsible for building muscle and expediating development and cell replication. It regulates the rejuvenation of muscle tissue.

When we are young, and our bodies are growing rapidly, we require a lot of protein and amino acids to keep up with cell replication and muscle development. Our bones are growing. Our hormones are on fire. We need a lot of fuel to stoke the fire and to keep us strong and healthy. We can eat pretty much whatever we want, and we seem to burn calories at the speed of a bullet train.

So, what is mTOR and how does it factor into the equation?

mTOR exists in every cell in the human body. mTOR controls many of our metabolic functions, not just muscle reproduction. It is constantly balancing and regulating our bodies. mTOR's job is to bring the body into homeostasis. It regulates our metabolism based on our protein, amino acid, and carbohydrate intake. mTOR is also responsible for regulating many of our growth hormones.

mTOR is responsible for rapid cell production and it feeds on the fuel from our diet. This fuel is primarily the protein we consume. mTOR is activated when we consume large amounts of animal proteins (or plant-based protein). It is also activated when we engage in rapid cardiovascular exercise.

There are two schools of thought on the mTOR debate. The first is that mTOR is an essential building block for cell replication and development. And that without it, we would become frail and age quickly.

The other is that mTOR serves a very important purpose as we are growing and developing, and it is unnecessary in high amounts as we get older. The diet we could get away with eating in our youth does not serve us well as we enter the later stages of our lives. Ever fed a teenager? They can eat milkshakes, burgers, salads, chips, tacos, pasta and still be hungry.

The reason for this is that their cell replication is highly active. They are growing and developing. If we tried to eat this way in our 40's, 50's or 60's and beyond, the result would be catastrophic, and we probably wouldn't be around that long.

A 2014 study published in 'Cell Metabolism' stated that, 'Respondents aged 50–65 reporting high protein intake had a 75% increase in overall mortality and a 4-fold increase in cancer death risk during the following 18 years. These associations were either abolished or attenuated if the proteins were plant derived.'**

**Reduction in IGF-1, Cancer, and Overall Mortality in the 65 and Younger but Not Older Population." Cell Metabolism, vol. 19, no. 3, Mar. 2014, pp. 407–17. www.cell.com, doi:10.1016/j.cmet.2014.02.006.

So how do we reduce mTOR as we get older? We can most definitely benefit from eating a plant-based diet. But for many people this is not entirely appetizing or sustainable. So how about committing to plant based for 70% or 80% of our meals? Sounds easy right? Well, the great news is – IT IS!

Having 3 or 4 days a week where we eat entirely plant based is attainable. Start with a diet model of Monday – Wednesday being 100% plant-based meals. As we all tend to enjoy a meal out or a splurge day, schedule these on your non-plant-based days. You could even start with one or two plant-based days. Plan out what you will eat. And remember, these are days when you are NOT going to track calories, carbohydrates, or any metrics you might ordinarily use.

Are you craving a burger – eat a plant based one. Pasta with a cream sauce? Substitute cashew cream. Swap the meat for mushrooms or lentils. I make a fabulous Bolognese pasta sauce using lentils and finely chopped mushrooms. Its delicious.

I am not saying that you should go bananas and eat in a way that is unhealthy. Try to include lots of fruit and vegetables in your plant-based daily intake. And if you want to go bananas then eat bananas. Bananas are a perfect food! Just remember not to combine them with meat and dairy.

Some health gurus even recommend dedicating a whole day to eating only fruits. Yes, an entire day. The main issue with eating fruit for an entire day is that you need to eat a lot of them to feel satiated. A common mistake is that people eat only one apple and then feel hungry in an hour. You need to eat a large quantity of fruit to feel full.

Ever felt particularly lethargic on a Monday? Perhaps you consumed too much of the wrong foods and possibly a few alcoholic beverages over the weekend? Well, Monday would be a perfect day to dedicate to eating fruit or plant based entirely. This gives your body a chance to pass the excess food and toxins through the digestive tract.

mTOR aids in helping us to grow and develop rapidly, but as we age, mTOR can actually become our worst enemy. Because it triggers massive cell replication, the waste cells can cause havoc if they are not removed from the body fast enough. The process of removing these cells is called Autophagy and we will touch on this later in the fasting Chapter.

mTor can trigger the replication of cancer cells and tumors. We only need 25-40 grams of protein per day, according to many doctors and nutritionists. Our Western diet often provides us with 80-150 grams of animal protein per day. This is excessive and it causes the internal organs to work overtime to rid the body of excess protein.

Let's face it... we are not all bodybuilders getting ready to go to the Olympics, right?

And even if we are, there are many plant-based alternatives that will provide us with cleaner, better protein options than meat and dairy.

THE SNEAKY AF* DIET BOOK

Chapter 5
High Protein Diets – The Myth

THE ANIMAL WAY				THE PLANT WAY			
HAKE	SIRLION STEAK	TUNA (CANNED)	CHICKEN THIGH (SKINLESS)	TEMPEH	TOFU	PUMPKIN SEEDS	AMARANTH (COOKED)
22g	24g	23g	28g	20g	8g	24g	4g
SALMON	CHICKEN BREAST	EGGS	LAMB CHOPS	LENTILS (COOKED)	KIDNEY BEANS	NUTRITIONAL YEAST	CHICKPEAS
20g	32g	13g	17g	8g	7g	51g	7g
LEAN PORK STEAK	10% (Fat) BEEF MINCE	PORK SAUSAGES	FILLET STEAK	TVP	QUINOA (COOKED)	EDAMAME	BUCKWHEAT
22g	28g	11g	21g	36g	5g	12g	8g
RIB EYE STEAK	PRAWNS	SMOKED SALMON	STREAKY BACON	SOYA BEANS (COOKED)	SEITAN (COOKED)	HEMP SEEDS	BLACK BEANS
24g	15g	22g	15g	14g	28g	22g	8g

PROTEIN per 100g

The reason high protein diets don't work is because our bodies are actually designed to consume plant-based foods.

Carnivores don't chew like we humans! They have very stable jaws. They tear flesh and move their jaws from side to side.

THE SNEAKY AF* DIET BOOK

Their teeth are extremely sharp like steak knives! Humans, and other herbivores, have teeth designed to consume plant-based materials. We can move our jaws in a range of motions. Our flat back molars are designed to grind plant-based materials.

I remember during my brief vegan stage in my late 20's we had invited a couple out for dinner. They looked after my African Grey parrot in Laguna when I travelled overseas.

I remember Pete explaining to me at dinner about how we are not designed to eat a vegan diet since we don't chew the cud like cows do.

I figured he was a bit of an expert on the evolutionary development of species. He is a rescuer of animals and has helped protect the migratory path of whales on their way to the Sea of Cortez to birth their calves. While I place absolutely no blame on him for this misinformation, I did switch to a meat-based diet shortly hereafter. I must say there was a part of my brain wanting to disbelieve this 'vegan' myth.

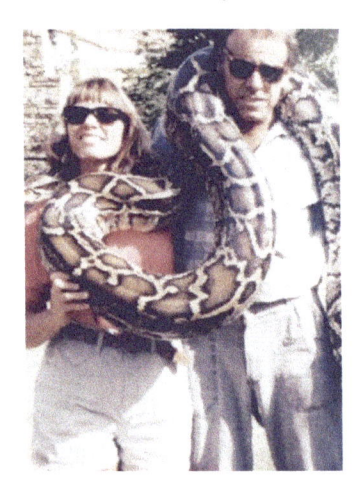

Pic: Pete & Libby

I had originally chosen to become a vegan because Jerry Corbetta had told me to read a book regarding the unfair slaughter practices of animals.

Once I had read this book, I couldn't unread it and the information was so disturbing that I decided to commit to a vegan diet.

Let me dispel a couple of myths here.

No, we do not need to chew the cud (like cows) to eat a vegan diet.

And we have incisors (teeth) designed to chew plant-based materials.

Some of the largest and strongest animals in the world consume plant-based diets.

At the time of writing this, I briefly heard that some Roman warriors had been unearthed. These were the strongest most bad-ass warriors. And guess what? Yep – they ate plant-based diets. Scientists could tell from their DNA that they ate a predominantly plant-based diet. Pretty amazing right?

We do not need animal protein to be strong and healthy.

Another fact that struck me was whilst watching a Netflix documentary on plant-based diets. A leading cardiologist was interviewed. He was saying that smoking is actually less harmful to you than eating a diet containing a high proportion of animal products.

What struck me in particular, was that he was discussing patients who adopted a keto diet and died in their 40's. Their friends and family would say 'They looked amazing', being unable to believe they had died.

Yes, they may have looked lean and fit on the outside but what was going on internally did not match their outer appearance.

Ever met a super-hot person and you think this is the one? Then you get to know them and realize they are cold and dark on the inside?

Well, it is sort of the same concept.

The average person only requires 10-40 grams of protein per day. The FDA recommends 40 grams of protein yet the average American eats 80-120 grams of protein per day. Meat and animal proteins, on average, take 12-14 hours to pass through the digestive tract.

Meat can wreak havoc on the digestive system as meat can turn toxic in the digestive tract, particularly when consumed with carbohydrates.

Urea is created by the body as a waste byproduct when too much protein is consumed. It is a nitrogenous end product of the metabolic process when excess protein is consumed by mammals. Yes, we are mammals! This results in putrefaction of the colon. (Imagine rotting meat in your colon… Ick!)

Proteins are made up of amino acids. Our body utilizes around 22 amino acids from proteins. Our body cannot produce 9 of these amino acids and they are called essential amino acids. When the excess amino acids are broken down, they are converted to ammonia which is toxic to the body, especially the liver and kidneys.

Plant proteins are often more balanced. They naturally contain carbohydrates and fiber, so they move through the colon more rapidly. Interestingly, plant proteins are treated quite differently by the body than animal proteins.

Plant-based proteins are much higher in glutamic acid. This is great for lowering your blood pressure. People who eat more meat typically have far higher cholesterol levels and blood pressure due to a buildup of plaque and a hardening of the arteries.

Eating animal protein can destroy the microbiome in the gut, leading to less effective digestion and discomfort after eating. In the 70's and 80's we looked up to Arnold Schwarzenegger, the amazing body builder, believing that we needed animal protein to gain muscle mass. Now he's a vegan! If you haven't watched The Game Changers, it's a must-see documentary.

There are too many facts to mention here and because I am writing this book to entertain you and hopefully transform you – I will not bore you with the details.

Do your own research. You'll see.

THE SNEAKY AF* DIET BOOK

Chapter 6
Water Consumption

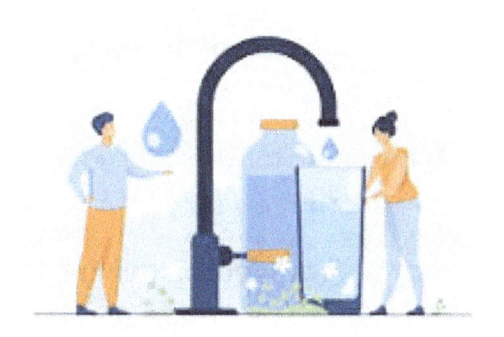

A great rule of thumb is to drink 5-6 large glasses of water per day. It seems like a lot, but I find if I drink water between meals, it is rather easy to consume this much water.

Water does a number of amazing things for the body. Water can help you to feel less hungry. Water removes waste and toxins from the body. Water helps to cleanse our internal organs. It lubricates tissues and joints.

Water is most essential to your overall health and wellness. Depending on where you live, your tap water may or may not be acceptable to drink.

It is not a bad idea to consider a water filtration system. These can range from a simple Brita jug that filters out contaminants to a more elaborate multi-filtration system that delivers amazing drinking water and is installed under your sink.

These have become much more affordable over the years.

Many of us skip the glass of water to consume soda or fruit juice.

Here's my rule of thumb.

Between meals I drink water.

With meals I drink tea, coffee, beer or wine (depending on what time of the day it is of course!).

The reason for this is that water can weaken digestive enzymes. A simple unsweetened iced tea would be a far better choice.

Another rule I live by is if I am feeling hungry, I stop and drink a full glass of filtered water. I wait around 20 minutes.

Often, I find I was not hungry at all. I was simply thirsty.

Many of us are dehydrated on a daily basis. Excessive caffeine consumption can trigger this. It is important to take the time to really consider how many glasses of water do we consume in a day. A good rule of thumb is a minimum of 6

 glasses of water to keep your body hydrated.

Here are some amazing things that will happen if you drink 6 - 8 glasses of water per day:

- You will feel hungry less often. Hunger is often just dehydration in disguise

- Drinking water will help to eliminate toxins from the body – your internal organs will function much better

- Water helps you to get the best out of your exercise regime – it keeps connective tissue and joints lubricated

- Water is a fat burner – without it you cannot effectively metabolize fat; a process called lipolysis

- Water is calorie free – ever count up the number of calories in sports drinks, sodas, blended coffees and other drinks?

- Increasing your water intake can speed up your metabolism

- Your hair and skin will look amazing – increases water intake has been linked to plumper skin cells make your skin glow!

One last note on water – buy a lovely refillable water bottle. Decorate it if you like! Buy a fancy one where you can add fruit to enhance the flavor.

Try not to buy plastic water bottles and the reason for this is twofold.

Firstly, many water companies do not use BPA approved plastic in the production of their mass-marketing cases of water.

These bottles are often shipped thousands of miles. If the water has a chance to heat up, often the contaminants in the plastic can leach into the water which is not healthy.

And secondly, you guessed it (I hope!) It is not good for the environment. Think of all of the 100's of millions of plastic bottles going into landfills each year. We cannot change this. But change begins with us – and our sphere of influence. And yes, I nag my friends about this one incessantly every time they try to hand me a plastic store bought water bottle.

Chapter 7
Is Sugar Good or Bad for my health?

Sugar has long been villainized and referred to as the main cause of Diabetes.

Let's break this down for you….

Many medical Doctors and nutritionists now realize that sugar is not the true issue. It is the lining of animal fat which coats the intestines making it impossible for the body to effectively absorb the sugar into the body and convert it into glucose. The glucose is then expended as energy.

If your intestines are coated in animal fat you cannot effectively absorb glucose.

Think about that. When you are eating an excessive amount of cheese and meat it is leaving a coating on your stomach and intestines.

This is making it very difficult for your body to not only absorb glucose but to absorb the nutrients from your food too.

Glucose is essential for fueling the body and the brain. Your body requires carbohydrates along with fat and protein to convert into fuel for the cells. Fat can be sourced from avocados, nuts, seeds and olives.

The brain relies almost entirely on glucose as its source of fuel. Ever heard anyone complaining about brain fog while on a high protein/low carb diet? Well, this is why.

The brain has no ability to store glucose, meaning it needs a constant supply of simple or complex carbohydrates which are then converted into glucose for the body and brain.

It is important to note that Complex Carbohydrates are a better source than Simple Carbohydrates.

Here is the difference:

EAT IN MODERATION: EAT MORE OF:

Simple	Complex
white bread, rice, and pasta	brown rice
candy	oats
soda	fruit
syrup	vegetables
table sugar	whole grains

All of the necessary protein and 'healthy' fats can be easily absorbed on a plant-based diet. Some of the largest strongest animals on the planet eat plant-based and are vegans.

Eat more grains, seeds, and nuts. Eat more fruit – a wonderful source of healthy sugar. Eat less refined sugars.

Chapter 8
Gut Health & Improving Your Microbiome

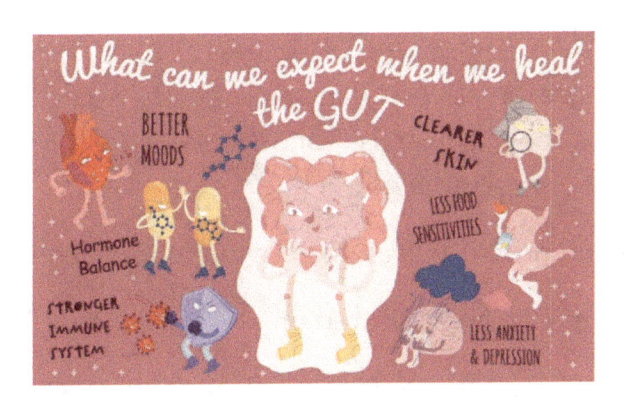

We have a second brain. A brain in our gut. Yes, it is true! It is often referred to as the Enteric Nervous System. It relies on the same type of neurons and neurotransmitters as our brain. It regulates hormones, blood flow and our immune system.

Our gut health has a profound effect on our mood and wellbeing. We have over one hundred trillion bacteria in the lower intestine and gut. Our immune cells line our gut. Maintaining a healthy microbiome is essential for fighting infections and staying healthy.

This has a profound effect on our neurotransmitters as many of these are creating in the stomach.

Maintaining a happy balance of gut flora is integral to feeling well and digesting food effectively. Flora refers to:

- Gut bacteria
- Intestinal flora
- Microbiota
- Microbiome
- Microflora

Antibiotics, preservatives, animal products, excessive alcohol, lack of sleep, lack of exercise, and stress can all interfere with healthy flora levels in the gut.

Prebiotics and probiotics can help to maintain healthy gut flora.

Whole books have been written on this topic alone.

An article, published in *Nature* publication in 2019, shows that eating red meat can drastically impact the gut microbiome in a negative manner.

'The old adage 'you are what you eat' could be extended to our gut microbiomes. Our diet shapes our gut microbiome by modulating the abundance of specific species and their individual or collective functions. Diet-induced changes in the gut microbiome could have important implications for host health as alterations in microbial functions affect host physiology and disease.'

Dairy can also have a dire impact on gut health. Although when these foods are eaten in a limited or sparingly way, we can maintain a healthy digestive system.

The great news is that these necessary prebiotics and probiotics can be provided from our diet. No need to go out and spend $40 on probiotics that often die in the gut.

Here are some ways to naturally maintain good gut flora.

1. Drink Kombucha! (In addition to the 6 – 8 glasses of water a day!)
   It's actually delicious. Choose a low sugar, refrigerated Kombucha. I drink a shot of lemon/ginger kombucha in the morning as soon as I wake up. For me it has a two-fold effect. It takes away my appetite for around an hour. And it helps my body to balance good gut flora naturally. I will often drink a shot of kombucha if I have eaten a heavy meal. I used to spend around $50 each month on refrigerated Probiotics and Prebiotics, until I watched an interesting podcast. A doctor explained that they are mostly useless by the time they hit the gut.

2. Eat fermented foods like Sauerkraut, Kimchi, Miso, Apple Cider Vinegar, Sourdough. Kefir, Yoghurt and Cheese also contain healthy levels of gut bacteria. It is often advised to eat whole, unsweetened yoghurt when on antibiotics as yoghurt can replenish much of the good bacteria in the gut which gets killed off by antibiotics.

3. Eat lots of legumes, vegetables, fruits, beans, nuts and seeds. Plant based can be delicious and super nutritious. It just takes a little more preparation and planning, but I promise you it is 100% worth it.

4. Eat a diet rich in Polyphenols like: grapes, green tea, almonds, blueberries, green leafy vegetables, and two of my favorites: red wine and dark chocolate.

5. Eat more whole grains! The western diet has become low in fiber. Fiber is essential to healthy gut flora. Instead of being absorbed by the small intestines, whole grains make their way to the large intestines where they promote the growth of healthy gut flora. Brown, red or black rice are excellent whole grains. Faro, oats, millet, barley, whole grain bread, popcorn and quinoa are all excellent. They can help to lower cholesterol, blood pressure and lower and stabilize insulin levels.

6. Eat a predominantly Plant Based Diet! Yes, it's that easy – eating completely plant based several days per week can help to promote good gut health. How? Meat and dairy negatively impact gut microbiomes. They also create inflammation and can lead to an increase of bacteria in the gut. Inflammation is the root cause of many illnesses. Keeping inflammation low in the body is key to great health. Plant based foods are high in beneficial good bacteria for the gut and animal-based products are high in bad bacteria.

7. Choose organic fruit and vegetables! There is a direct correlation between soil-based probiotics (SBO's) and good gut health. Many of the fruits and vegetables we consume are grown in bad soil and sprayed with numerous pesticides. This in turn affects our gut flora.

Eating organic ensures that we can absorb nutrients from the food we eat. Eat a rainbow of colors! *(This does not mean skittles).*

8. Drink coffee and tea! They are full of polyphenols and antioxidants. This is a way healthier drink than fruit juice which is often high in sugar and has the essential necessary fiber removed.

9. My favorite! Eat dark chocolate! It is a wonderful and delicious treat. It is not only high in polyphenols, but it also contains high levels of flavanols and catechins.

10. Avoid ultra processed foods. Cut out any fake sugars and preservatives wherever possible. The body does not know what to do with fake sugars and can store them as fat cells. Choose brown sugar, coconut sugar, maple syrup or even honey as a sweetener. Honey is not considered vegan. However, it is not something I have cut out of my diet as I love honey! I try to buy honey from a farmers' market whenever possible.

THE SNEAKY AF* DIET BOOK

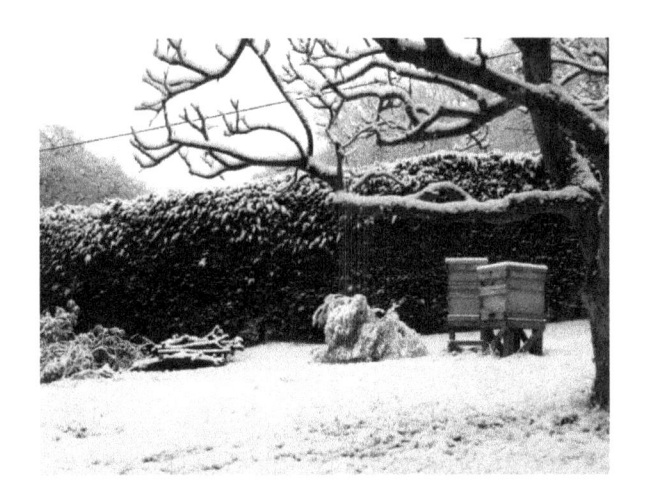

My bee hives in the UK!

Chapter 9
You Can Help the Environment

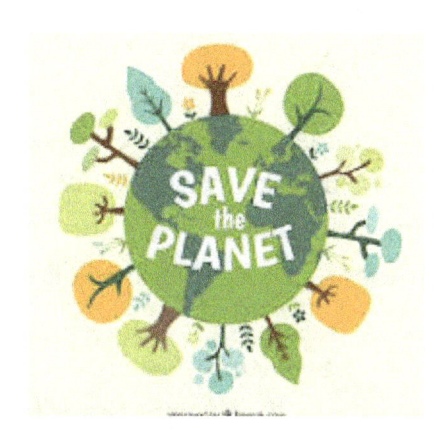

With more than 83 billion animals reared and slaughtered globally for the food industry every year, industrial scale animal agriculture impacts our environment in an enormously detrimental way.

It is not only one of the leading contributors to climate change and deforestation, but it also uses vast quantities of water. Research shows that switching to more plant-forward diets could cut our negative climate footprint in half, so by changing our diet to reduce or replace meat, dairy and eggs with more water-friendly plant-based foods, we can all help to preserve the world's water.

THE SNEAKY AF* DIET BOOK

1. Farming (animal and plant) accounts for about 70 percent of water used in the world today, up to 92 percent of freshwater, with nearly one-third of that related to animal farming and growing crops to feed to animals.

2. Most of the total volume of water used for animal agriculture (98 percent) refers to the water footprint of the feed for the animals. About one-third of the world's grain and 80 percent of the world's soy is fed to the animals we rear for food.

3. Intensive animal farming can cause serious water pollution such as eutrophication, an excessive amount of algae in the water caused by run-off of animal feces and leftover feed, often leading to loss of fish and other aquatic wildlife.

4. 725.6L of fresh water are needed to produce 100g of protein from beef, whereas tofu requires eight times less freshwater (92.9L)

5. 96 percent of fish eaten in Europe comes from fresh-water fish farming, but the vast quantities of fish excrement and uneaten fish food that settles on the pond bed make the perfect and awful environment for the production of the greenhouse gas methane.

6. A meat-free diet can cut our water footprint in half! Studies show that a healthy meat-free diet reduces our water footprint by up to 55%.

7. The United Nations Environment Assembly says that plant-

based burgers require between 75 – 99 percent less water; 93 – 95 per cent less land; and generate 87 – 90 per cent fewer emissions than regular beef burgers.

8. *"A vegan diet is probably the single biggest way to reduce your impact on planet Earth, not just greenhouse gases, but global acidification, eutrophication, land use and water use. It is far bigger than cutting down on your flights or buying an electric car,"* said University of Oxford's Joseph Poore, who led the most comprehensive analysis on the damage farming does to the planet.

Go plant based for the animals and the environment – if that's what motivates you. Or just to shed some pounds and feel great.

We are experiencing a climate catastrophe. The planet's temperature is increasing. It will render many parts of the earth uninhabitable over the next 10-20 years.

Dairy farming and animal and meat production is one of the biggest contributors to rapid climate change.

The great news is that you can help. Just by decreasing your intake of dairy and meat you can help to make the earth's surface more carbon dynamic. Notice – I used the word 'decrease'. I am not advocating that you cut out any of the foods you love altogether. I am only suggesting that you dedicate a few days a week to eating plant-based foods.

Sustainable farming of fruit and vegetables helps to absorb carbon. Choosing organic reduces the number of pesticides and harmful chemicals used in the cultivation of the food we consume.

Your choice to opt for plant-based foods will help force companies to pivot and diversify. The higher the demand for organic produce and plant-based alternatives, the more farmers will provide what is in demand. Eventually it is reflected in a lower price of organic produce as more and more farmers shift to meet supply.

We cannot continue to rape and pillage the planet without some form of backlash from mother nature (Aya). Whether it be natural disasters, disease, food famines or the like. We are already seeing these global catastrophes in epic proportions. It is only going to get worse if we continue on this path. If we continue there will not be a planet for our grandchildren and our great grandchildren.

Earth will survive and adapt. It has done so for billions of years. But humans, as a species, may not survive. I know this sounds extreme, but it is happening before our very eyes. And you can be a precursor to positive change, just by starting a plant-based diet! It can and will have a profound effect on the planet and the generations to come.

Chapter 10
The Scientific Evidence Is Overwhelming

Dr Michael Greger explains, *"After a meal of animal products people suffer from endotoxemia, their blood stream becomes awash with bacterial toxins known as endotoxins that are present in the animal products, no wonder our body goes crazy"*.

-Taken from LiveKindly 'Health & Wellness'

So, what exactly is Endotoxemia?

The term endotoxemia refers to a high concentration of toxins in your blood cells. In other words, it is a toxic overload in your body's 'cells. And the root cause of endotoxemia, and many other health conditions for that matter, lies in the microbiome or 'gut'.

You've probably heard of leaky gut, where the gastrointestinal lining has issues with increased permeability allowing particles to flow into the bloodstream. These are particles, bacteria and waste and antigens, like undigested food proteins that have no business being there. One particle in particular that is causing a lot of trouble – these are called lipopolysaccharides or LPS.

THE SNEAKY AF* DIET BOOK

Lipopolysaccharides (LPS) are large complex molecules found in gram-negative bacteria. LPS are endotoxins and when absorbed they can cause a very strong overreaction of the immune system.

I am not a scientist. But I do trust in clinical trials and data.

- 100 million Americans have Type II Diabetes or are pre diabetic

- 40% of Americans over 50 years of age are obese

- The only source of artery blocking cholesterol is animal derived

- A plant-based diet can easily reverse heart disease and Type II diabetes within a few months

- Heart Disease is the No.1 cause of death in America

- The USA government works closely with the meat and dairy industry as do many of the charities. They promote and subsidize these products. *What the actual fuck! They are out to kill us!*

- Many cancers can now be attributed to diet (90%) And, surprisingly only 10% is genetic
  'Animal protein, unlike plant protein, causes the body to produce higher levels of the hormone IGF-Excessive production of this hormone is linked to the growth of certain cancers.' **

** https://oopsvegan.com/en/blog/veganism-and-health

Many of the scientific studies show a clear correlation between longevity and a predominantly plant-based diet. There are some studies that contradict this notion, but they are limited.

A few places in the world are called "Blue Zones." The term refers to *'geographic areas in which people have low rates of chronic disease and live longer than anywhere else'*.

When we look at areas called 'Blue Zones' where people live well into their 100's and beyond, one defining characteristic is that these people eat a high proportion of plant-based foods and a low proportion of animal products.

I visited Vilcabamba in Ecuador with the intention of purchasing a vacation home there. My chiropractor had told me that they had established a Longevity Centre to research why people lived over 100 years old and often to their 120th birthday and beyond.

I was fascinated by this information.

I booked my trip. Well, firstly I booked a seminar on International Living in Las Vegas scheduled for a few months out.

Then I booked my airfare to Ecuador leaving the following week. Because I am spontaneous like that. Possibly a bit stupid too.

THE SNEAKY AF* DIET BOOK

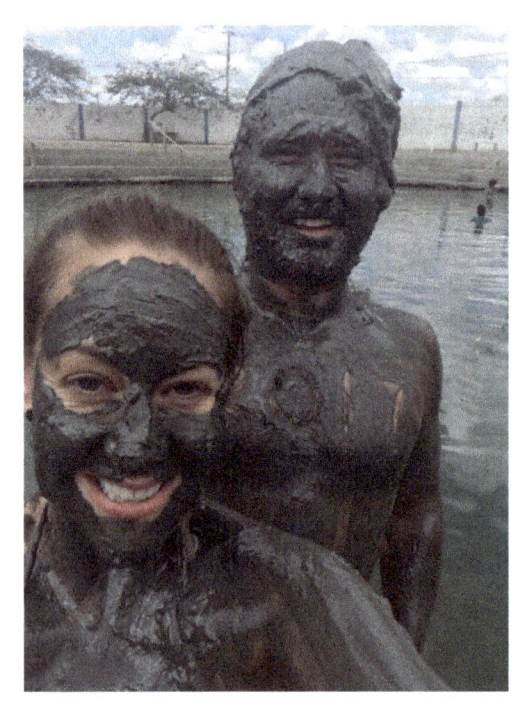

A few things happened during that vacation.

I met some wonderful people. Quito was amazing. Vilcabamba was a tiny little magical town. I figured it was a little too slow paced for me though. I did learn one of the reasons for longevity is the unusually high occurrence of negative ions in the valley. The food was wonderful. The beer tasted great.

Picture: Santa Elena mud baths, Ecuador

Another reason is that their main source of drinking water is very high in minerals and colloidal silver. It is largely untreated and is tapped from an underground source.

The inhabitants eat a primarily plant-based diet and

 very low in animal fat. They eat predominantly grains, legumes and fresh vegetables with some freshwater fish and meat occasionally.

Another fascinating aspect of this sacred valley is that the inhabitants often exercise at 5am or 6am. It is not uncommon to see groups of local elders exercising in the main square.

This is a common aspect of these blue zones around the world. Clean, predominantly plant-based diet, exercise and lack of processed foods.

I loved Vilcabamba, but it was rather quiet and rural. I enjoyed some fabulous food and I met some lovely people.

However, I decided to set off for the coast. I love the beach. I had heard there was a great coastal town full of ex-pats from all over the world. I arrived in Salinas and enjoyed a fabulous meal. I asked the waiter for a recommendation on a hotel. He suggested a lovely hotel with a casino. Very Vegas

I did learn that I should not be so trusting of people when I travel (and yes, I have learned this lesson previously) especially as a single woman travelling alone. I learned that possibly I should not go back to a gated compound with a man I met in casino who had two bodyguards. Too much wine can impair my judgement on occasion.

Fortunately, I pulled the 'poor me' card when he asked if any of my relatives had money to pay a ransom. He was pretty loaded (and I don't mean wealthy). I explained to him that my father had cancer and I did lots of great things for charity. He certainly wouldn't want to kidnap little old me.

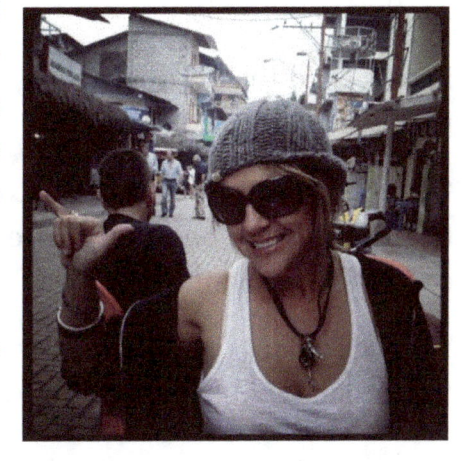

After a little more discussion and limited visible panic on my side (trust me, I was feeling extremely panicked

internally), he had one of the bodyguards drive me back to my hotel. In my defense, he was rather hot and had been a male model in Miami.

In any case, I returned to America. Two weeks later I bought a house, sight unseen, in a wonderful little town called Olon. I have many happy and wonderful memories of visiting Ecuador.

Their diet is simple. The food is delicious. They eat plantains and rice with most meals. The seafood is locally caught in the morning. The grocery stores are sparse as most of the food is fresh.

It is relatively hard to find processed food in Ecuador. Somehow, a few weeks' vacation in Ecuador would always leave me feeling revitalized and renewed and I believe a large portion of this equation is that the food was so simple yet wonderful.

I finally concluded I could not possibly retire in Ecuador as I would miss the modern luxuries we take for granted in the USA. And I'd miss Trader Joes too much, so I settled back into life in Southern California.

I finally sold the house after 8 years of memorable vacations. I highly recommend Ecuador.

One of my most memorable vacations was taking my mother to Ecuador. I have been fortunate enough to take her to many countries around the world.

We checked into an Airbnb in Banos and the sweet gal who ran the Airbnb (unbeknownst to us) had set up quite the itinerary. I don't think she understood my mother was in her 70's. She certainly doesn't look it.

She sent us off to go white water rafting and the day after, she sent us ziplining. Being somewhat of an adrenaline junkie (dopamine give me more – more about that in a later chapter), I relished the idea of ziplining.

This was probably my 10th time ziplining, but nothing prepared me for this experience. It was truly terrifying. But exciting too.

Mainly I was terrified for my 70-year-old mother.

I had actually threatened the guide during white water rafting the day before, not to overturn the boat under any circumstance. Mainly because my mother was on board. And we were in the middle of a rather large river with boulders and No.3 rapids.

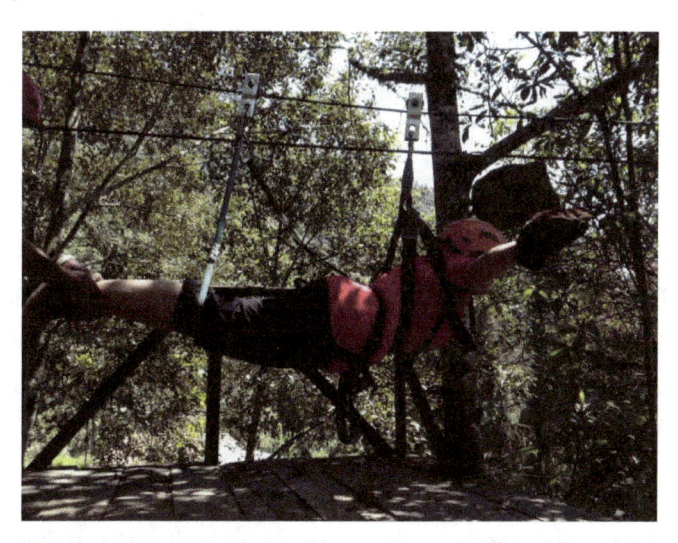

Mum got through the ziplining experience. And yes, she has travelled with me since. A safer alternative. A Holland America cruise to Alaska. For illustration purposes here is a photo of mum preparing to zipline. I purposefully chose a photo which obscured her face so you cannot see how truly terrified she was.

I digress….

Back to the Scientific Evidence of Eating Plant-Based!

How long does it take to reverse a lifetime of meat and dairy eating? Here is a timeline of changes after you start eating plant-based:

1 - 3 hours – Your insulin levels will stabilize. Eating fruits, vegetables and wholegrains will lower any spikes in insulin, helping you to feel less hungry.

Day 3 – 6 – Your energy will improve. You will start sleeping better. You will go to the bathroom more regularly as you will be eating a higher fiber diet with less meat and dairy to clog the intestines.

Week 1 -2 – Your cholesterol will have become lower. Multiple studies and documentaries have documented this change via bloodwork. The great news is that many people dependent on Statins and other cholesterol medications are able to adjust their medication *(with a doctor's supervision of course!)*. Your blood pressure will most probably have decreased too!

Week 2 - 3 *(and beyond)* – You will most probably see a marked decrease in weight specifically around the belly, things and upper arms. It's important to avoid high sugar and high fat foods. There is such a thing as a junk food vegan! Providing you stick to whole grain foods, fruits and vegetables, and healthy non processed foods you will be fine.

Week 3 - 4 – Food will begin to taste better. Most of us are so used to salty, sugary processed food that at first, plant-based food may taste a bit boring. But hang in there. As you begin to restore your taste buds you will find you will crave healthy delicious food. And the thought of salty, greasy bacon will turn your stomach.

Month 1 – 2 – Your skin will appear most supply. It will take on a glow. Many teenagers find that acne and skin issues clear up completely on a plant-based diet. Another wonderful side effect is that eating plant based can be great for your sex life. Just watch the amazing documentary *'The Game Changers'*, for scientific proof on this one.

Month 2 – 6 – Better sleep! More energy! Looking slim and healthy! Your arteries will have become cleaner. The only source of cholesterol is animal fat or unhealthy oil. If you have eliminated these from your diet you will have successfully improved blood circulation throughout the body and lowered your chance of a stroke or heart attack.

Heart disease and cardiovascular disease are the number one killer worldwide.

A few fun facts:

'Most studies clearly show that consuming a more plant-based diet is much healthier than a diet high in animal protein. There are some studies claiming that high meat intake is not unhealthy, but they are

significantly in the minority; the scientific evidence is overwhelmingly in favor of a more plant-based diet instead of a high-animal-protein diet. '

'Growing evidence suggests potential cardiovascular benefits of plant-based diets and dietary patterns, defined as a dietary profile, which emphasizes the high intake of plant-based food products while limiting the intake of animal products. Higher consumption of plant foods has been shown to reduce systolic blood pressure and plasma triglyceride levels, thereby exerting protective effects against obesity and incident diabetes. Besides reducing CVD risk factors, previous studies have also indicated an association between plant-based diets and improved quality of life, such as an improved quality of sleep, reduced likelihood of mental health disorders, and decreased rate of cognitive decline.'**

**https://www.ncbi.nlm.nih.gov/pmc/articles/PMC8604150/

The Association of Plant Based Diet With Cardiocvascular Disease and Mortality

Chapter 11
Become a Flexitarian!

I do get teased a lot by my friends for being a 'part-time vegan'. They wonder why I'll eat a steak (occasionally) or try some cheese at a party.

What they don't see is that most of my days are plant-based. When left to my own devices I will choose vegan foods. I will make myself vegan meals.

I will buy vegan ingredients at the grocery store. I will find vegan alternatives to the foods I love.

I will research vegan recipes that mimic (and often taste better than) their meat and dairy based old favorites.

Really, I'm a flexitarian. I love this term. I'm not vegan. I'm not an 100% plant-based eater. I eat what my body craves *(only when I truly crave something)* and the rest of the time I eat a clean and healthy diet filled with fruits, vegetables, whole grains, nuts and seeds.

There are many iterations of vege-eaters out in the world!

Vegetarian: Also known as the ovo-lactovegetarian, this diet includes all plant-based foods. It also allows for eggs and dairy. Much of Southern India fit into this category.

Vegan: This is a diet that consists of plant-based foods. It excludes all meat, dairy, and eggs. Many vegans choose not to eat honey. Many people who follow this diet do so for ethical or environmental reasons.

Pescatarian: This is a largely vegetarian diet that includes all plant-based foods and sometimes dairy. Pescatarians eat seafood as their predominant source of protein.

Whole-foods & plant-based: Most like a vegan diet, this diet focuses on the health benefits of eliminating meat and dairy. It is a diet laden with fruit, vegetables and whole grains while low in fat.

***Flexetarian:** This is a broad term used by those who primarily follow a vegan or a plant-based diet, but allow for some meat, dairy, and seafood on occasion.*

Allowing flexibility in your diet means that you will never get bored of eating a certain way.

If someone told me, I could never eat a slice of cake or a donut again I would feel rather sad.

Would I eat these foods every day? No.

On a special occasion? Yes!

Life and diet do not have to be all or nothing. Maintaining a healthy balance is key. I find the healthier the food I eat – the better I feel.

The more plant-based foods I eat the more often I get out of the shower and catch a glimpse of myself in the mirror and think wow! I look slim. I feel great. And it encourages me to adopt this way of eating for most of my life.

But that slice of birthday cake at a friend's party? I am going to say yes to that. And I feel I can as it only makes up a small proportion of my food intake.

You can have your cake and eat it too!

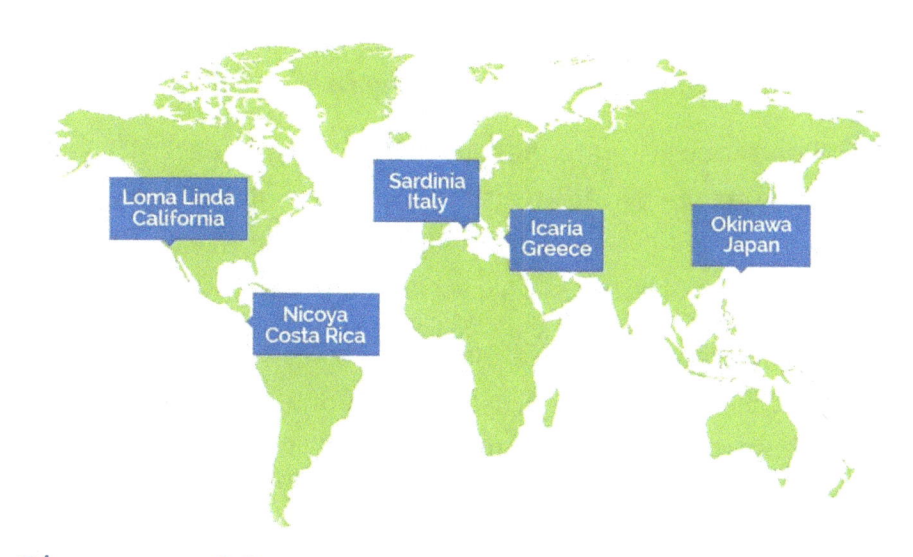

Chapter 12
Blue Zones

There are currently 5 recognized Blue Zones around the world. What are Blue Zones? Blue Zones are areas of the world where people live the longest lives, consistently reaching age 100. In contrast, the average life expectancy in the U.S. is currently 77 years, according to the CDC.

People in Blue Zones all seem to have a few things in common. They eat a diet of primarily plant-based foods. They restrict sugars and processed foods. They eat smaller amounts more often. They eat a diet rich in fruits, vegetables, and grains. And they exercise daily.

It is estimated that children in the USA will have shorter life expectancies than their parents, due to bad diet choices and lack of exercise. Thirty years ago, over 60% of children walked to school. Today, only around 12% of children walk to school. It's no wonder childhood obesity is on the rise.

Childhood obesity rate has tripled over the past 40 years. According to the World Health Organization, 42 million children under the age of five were overweight or obese around the world in 2013. This number has only accelerated since then.

British celebrity chef, Jamie Oliver, has started several programs to help children eat healthier foods. In 2009, they measured the success of banning soft drinks, providing more fruit and vegetables, and restricting fried foods in schools. The report was conducted by the Institute of Social and Economic Research at Essex University, UK.

The research was conducted on 11-year-old children. They allowed a full year for the results to be measured. Science test scores increased by 8% and English test scores by 6%, purely from a change in diet.

The research conducted on Blue Zones has shown that these centurions (people who live over the age of 100), eat primarily grains, fruits and vegetables.

Loma Linda, California

LOMA LINDA, CALIFORNIA, US
HOW LOMA LINDA CENTENARIANS ATE FOR MOST OF THEIR LIVES

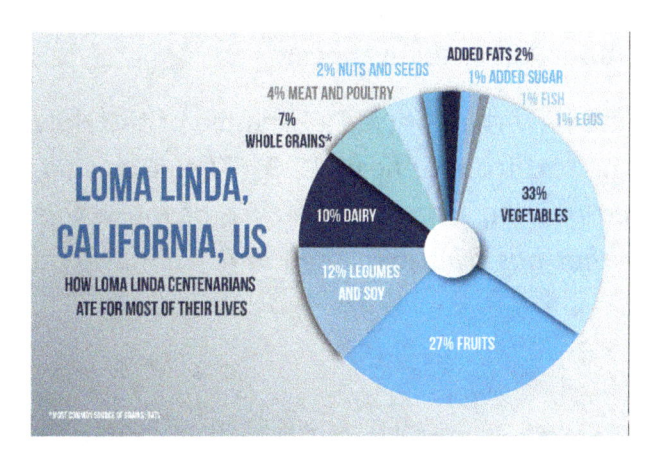

- 33% VEGETABLES
- 27% FRUITS
- 12% LEGUMES AND SOY
- 10% DAIRY
- 7% WHOLE GRAINS*
- 4% MEAT AND POULTRY
- 2% NUTS AND SEEDS
- ADDED FATS 2%
- 1% ADDED SUGAR
- 1% FISH
- 1% EGGS

Loma Linda, located in sunny California, is considered a Blue Zone due to its large population of Seventh Day Adventists and centenarians. They exercise regularly, consume a healthy diet with very little meat and dairy. They *(mostly)* do not drink or smoke.

Adventists who consume nuts at least 5 times per week have half the risk of heart disease (the number one killer in the world) than those who don't.

They also spend a lot of time with other Seventh Day Adventists and have a strong sense of community, a common theme in all Blue Zones.

They believe in smaller portions sizes. They also believe in eating breakfast like a king and reducing portion sizes later in the day.

THE SNEAKY AF* DIET BOOK

They support a Biblical diet of fruits, nuts and seeds. Adventists who ate legumes 3-4 times a week (such as beans, chickpeas and peas) had a 30 - 40% reduction in colon cancer.

Seventh Day Adventists view the body as a "Temple of the Holy Spirit". They rely on the text from Genesis 1:29: *"Then God said, "I give you every seed-bearing plant on the face of the whole earth and every tree that has fruit with seed in it. They will be yours for food."*

And here's a recipe from The Loma Linda University! Craving a healthy, sweet treat? Here it is! It's Gluten Free and Vegan!

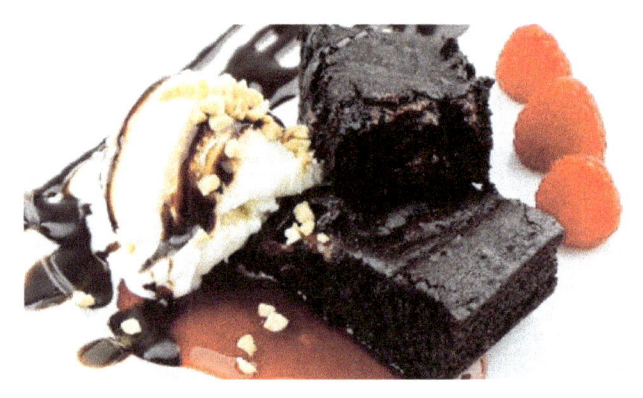

Recipe: Date Brownies

Servings per recipe: 5
Prep time: 15 minutes
Cook time: 25 minutes

INGREDIENTS

- 1 C Almond flour, blanched (or regular flour)
- 1 C Medjool dates, pitted and soaked in hot water
- 3 Eggs, large
- 1/4 C Raw honey (or sweetener of choice)
- 1/4 C Extra-virgin coconut oil, melted
- 1 tsp. Pure vanilla
- 1/2 C Dark cocoa powder
- 1/2 tsp. Cinnamon
- 1/2 tsp. Baking soda
- 1/4 tsp. Salt
- ¼ C Dark Chocolate chips

DIRECTIONS

A food processor works best to prepare these, but you can also use a stand mixer or hand mixer. If you use the latter, you will need to process the dates in a small food processor or chop them very finely before adding them to the batter.

Preheat oven to 350 degrees. Soak dates in hot water for 10 minutes. When draining, gently press out excess water. Place all ingredients (except for the eggs) in a large food processor and pulse for a minute or so until well combined. Be sure to check that there are no large pieces of unprocessed dates.

Add the eggs, one at a time, pulsing each time for about 30 seconds to thoroughly combine them into the batter.

Line a large baking dish (of choice, depending on desired thickness) with parchment paper then pour in the batter. Bake in the oven for about 25 minutes or until a toothpick inserted into the center comes out clean but somewhat moist. Remove the brownies immediately from the oven, let cool then cut into desired size. Store them in the fridge for up to 5 days. These are also freezer-friendly so make an extra batch and store some in the freezer.

Nicoya, Costa Rica

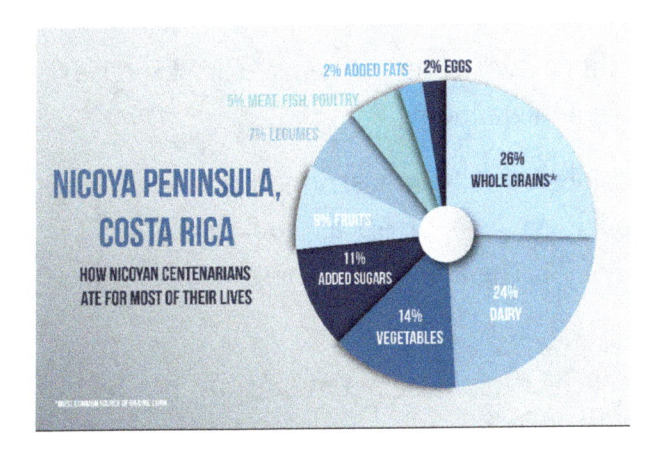

NICOYA PENINSULA, COSTA RICA
HOW NICOYAN CENTENARIANS ATE FOR MOST OF THEIR LIVES

- 2% ADDED FATS
- 2% EGGS
- 5% MEAT, FISH, POULTRY
- 7% LEGUMES
- 26% WHOLE GRAINS*
- 9% FRUITS
- 11% ADDED SUGARS
- 24% DAIRY
- 14% VEGETABLES

As you can see, the centenarians of Nicoya Peninsula eat a diet rich in whole grains and vegetables. Surprisingly, they do eat dairy, but most of the dairy they consume is non-processed.

They also have a wonderful sense of family and community. The elders spend time with neighbors, children and grandchildren.

They eat fewer calories which is surprisingly easy to do when eating a diet rich in fruits, vegetables and grains.

They enjoy spending 15-30 minutes in the sun each day ensuring they have a good intake of Vitamin D from the sun.

Another surprising fact is that they have a water supply that is considered 'hard water' meaning it is naturally high in calcium which promotes strong bones and teeth.

They live by a simple principle of finding one's purpose. The locals call it *'plan de vida'* which literally translates to *'soul's purpose'*.

THE SNEAKY AF* DIET BOOK

They feel a need to contribute to the greater good of the community, often lending a helping hand to those in need.

Many of the inhabitants have never driven a car. Exercise is integral to their lifestyle and wellbeing.

As of 2021, The Costa Rican health ministry had recorded more than 900 residents over the age of 90 as well as over 5,000 residents over the age of 75. The majority of these residents were in good health.

And now a delicious 'perfect' plant-based meal from the Nicoya Peninsula....

RECIPE : 5 MINUTE TASTY SQUASH AND BEANS

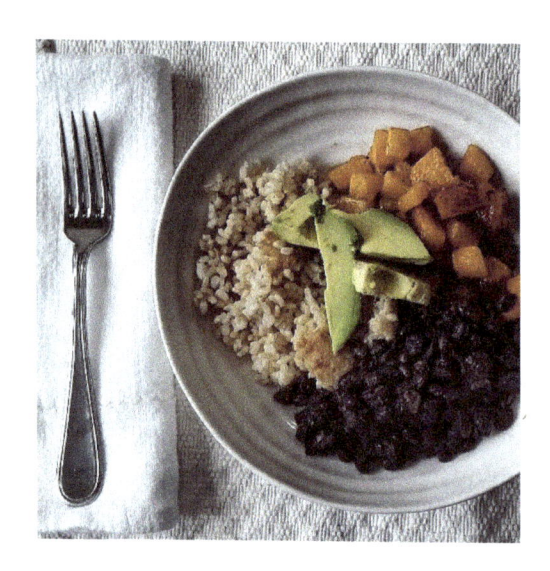

INGREDIENTS

- 1 cup black beans

- 1 cup of brown rice
- 1 large squash
- 1 avocado
- 4 T olive oil
- hot sauce of your choice
- dash of salt

DIRECTIONS

5-Minute Way

- 1 can of black beans
- 1 pouch of precooked brown rice (available at Trader Joe's)
- 1 bag of seeded, peeled and cubed squash, tossed lightly in olive oil
1. Microwave all ingredients in separate bowl until hot.
2. Serve together. Top with sliced avocado with a dash of hot sauce.

Slow Food Way

1. Soak beans overnight, rinse thoroughly and boil (add garlic if desired) for 50 minutes.
2. Peel and seed squash, dice into half-inch cubes and toss lightly in olive oil.
3. Place the squash on a cookie sheet and bake 350°F for 50 minutes.
4. Serve all hot ingredients together. Top with sliced avocado with a dash of hot sauce. Salt and pepper to taste.

Sardinia, Italy

SARDINIA, ITALY
HOW SARDINIAN CENTENARIANS ATE FOR MOST OF THEIR LIVES

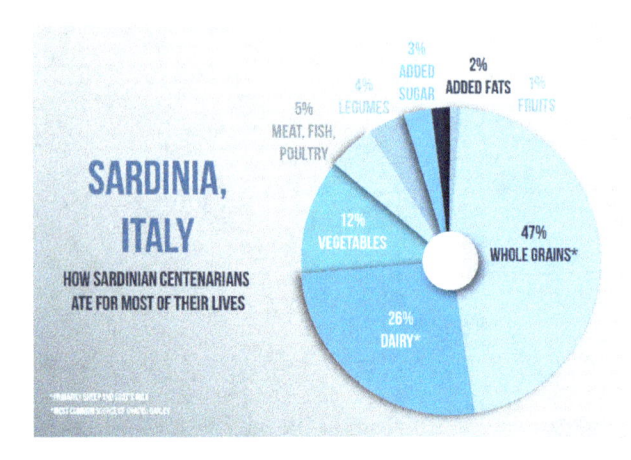

- 47% WHOLE GRAINS*
- 26% DAIRY*
- 12% VEGETABLES
- 5% MEAT, FISH, POULTRY
- 4% LEGUMES
- 3% ADDED SUGAR
- 2% ADDED FATS
- 1% FRUITS

Sardinia is a small kidney shaped island off the coast of Italy. It is comprised of many villages that seem to have stopped in time and remained as they would have been hundreds of years ago.

Sardinians spend their lives rather traditionally. They live close to friends and family and retain these relationships throughout their lives.

Their diet consists mainly of whole grains and the main source is barley which they grow themselves in their gardens.

They do consume dairy, but it is important to note that the source is not from cow's milk, it is primarily goat or sheep's milk.

They often hunt and fish for their meals.

Sardinians believe in enjoying a meal with friends and family and laughing over a glass or two of red wine. Their local wine varietal is *Grenache* (a delicious red) and it is high in antioxidants. It is not highly processed and is usually enjoyed 'young' which keeps the alcohol level to a minimum.

They exercise regularly and enjoy growing their own fruits and vegetables. Due to a lack of pesticides and a favorable climate, their food source is organic and healthy.

Many occupants do not drive so walking is their method of transportation. The terrain is rough and rugged ensuring low – medium impact exercise just to complete daily tasks.

THE SNEAKY AF* DIET BOOK

Now a delicious Sardian recipe:

Recipe: Sardinian Pasta Fagiole

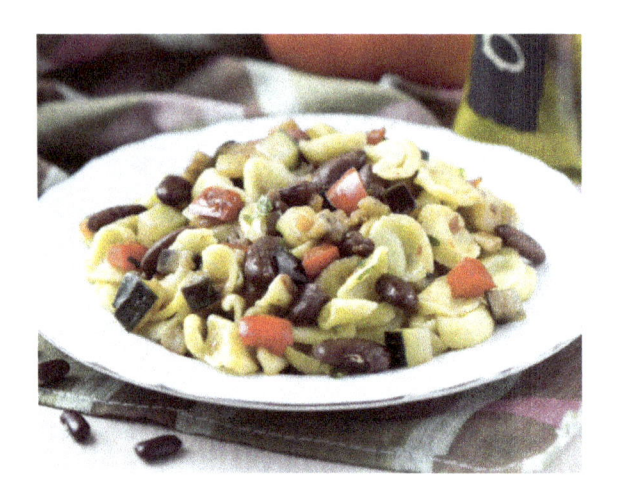

INGREDIENTS

- 1 large onions, chopped finely
- 1 lb great northern beans or navy beans (can use canned, wash well)
- 3 stalks fresh celery, finely diced
- 1 x cup of black olives (I prefer pitted)
- 1 cup chopped zucchini
- Fresh garlic or garlic powder to taste
- 1 x 8oz can whole tomatoes, chopped or diced, you can use 4 fresh tomatoes instead
- 1/2 cup flat Italian parsley, chopped
- 2-3 cups vegetable broth to start (can add more as it cooks down)
- 1/2 lb whole grain spaghetti or elbow pasta
- Splash of red wine

- Red pepper flakes (optional)
- Salt and pepper to taste
- 1/2 cup parmesan cheese (optional) You can use any vegan cheese or nutritional yeast which is high in B12

DIRECTIONS

If using dried beans:

1. Wash and soak beans for 2 hours, if using dried.
2. Rinse beans and bring to a boil with lid on pot. Don't let it boil over. Use at least 1/2 gallon of water. Cook until semi tender. (skip this step if using canned beans, just ensure to wash them well)
3. Add celery and onion to a large saucepan with a little olive oil on low heat. Fry these ingredients for around 15-20 minutes. Add garlic for the final 1-2 minutes. Add all other ingredients (including the beans but not the pasta) including vegetable broth, and cook over medium to high heat, stirring occasionally to avoid burning.
4. Continue to cook until the beans are tender (about 2-3 hours). Add broth as needed. Add the olives, red pepper flakes and salt and pepper in the final 10 minutes of cooking. You can add a tiny amount of flour mixed with water to thicken the sauce if desired.
5. Cook pasta separately in boiling salt water until al dente. Rinse, drain, and cool.
6. Mix the pasta and all ingredients, add a sprinkle of parmesan cheese (optional) and parsley, and serve hot.

Ikaria, Greece

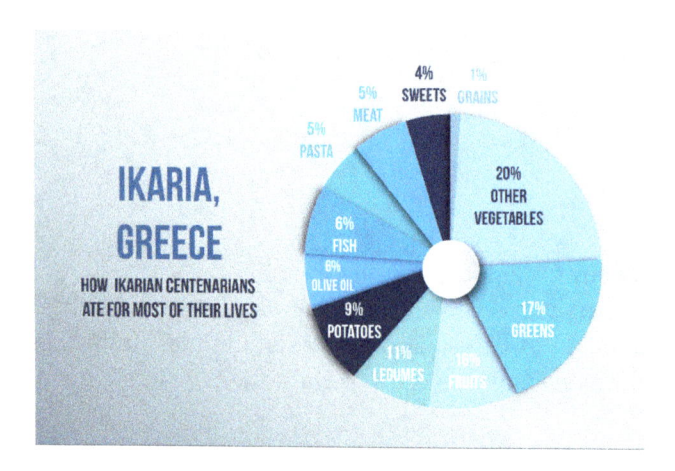

IKARIA, GREECE
HOW IKARIAN CENTENARIANS ATE FOR MOST OF THEIR LIVES

- 20% OTHER VEGETABLES
- 17% GREENS
- 13% FRUITS
- 11% LEGUMES
- 9% POTATOES
- 6% OLIVE OIL
- 6% FISH
- 5% PASTA
- 5% MEAT
- 4% SWEETS
- 1% GRAINS

One in three Ikarians make it to their 90's. Their culture and traditions have been steeped in family values.

They drink goat's milk instead of cow's milk which seems to be a theme amongst Blue Zones.

The majority of their food is unprocessed. They rely on local, in season produce. They predominantly eat fresh, locally sourced fruits, vegetables and plant-based foods.

They cook using locally sourced olive oil.

They nap regularly. It is little wonder with temperatures that can reach well into the 50's (Celsius). An afternoon siesta is a perfect way to escape the summer sun. It has been proven that people who nap more often have a far lower incidence of heart disease. This may be attributed to a lowered rate of stress.

The longest living Ikarians live in the mountainous regions. They get exercise by gardening or walking to a friend or relative's house which may involve a long uphill trek.

They often fast for religious reasons. They believe in eating smaller portions spread out during the day.

They regularly enjoy herbal tea with a friend regularly. This is a part of their social engagement. They value community and friendships and rarely spend time in isolation.

They have a strong sense of family and community, and they continue to garden of work on the land well into their later years. Stress and loneliness are almost nonexistent.

Many Ikarians do not have a phone or a television, and many rarely look at a clock. They rely on the sun.

A delicious Ikarian dish….

Ikarian Stuffed Eggplants

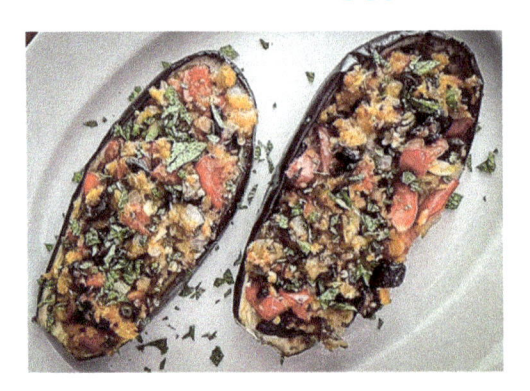

INGREDIENTS

- 3 medium eggplants, cut length ways, ends removed
- 1/4 cup parsley, chopped
- 2 large tomatoes, diced or 1 x 8oz can
- 1 onion, finely diced
- 3 cloves garlic, sliced finely
- 1/2 cup extra-virgin olive oil
- 1 sweet potato, peeled and cubed
- 1 bell pepper (green, red, or yellow), diced
- 1 tblsp capers, drained
- 1/3 cup of breadcrumbs (I like to grate my own using sour dough)
- Red Pepper Flakes (optional)
- Salt and pepper to taste

DIRECTIONS

1. Add a little olive oil to the front and back of the eggplants and season with salt and pepper.
2. Bake in the oven for 30 minutes.

3. Boil water in a saucepan and add the sweet potato cooking until tender (15 minutes)
4. Remove eggplant and wait to cool. Scoop out most of the inner part of the eggplant.
5. In a medium bowl, mix together parsley, tomatoes, and a few more teaspoons of olive oil as your stuffing mixture. Add eggplant and drained sweet potato.
6. In a separate pan, sauté onions and bell pepper for 8 - 10 minutes, or until tender. Add garlic for the last minute or two.
7. Combine all ingredients, tasting to see if it requires salt or pepper. Scoop the mixture into the eggplant skins. Top with breadcrumbs.
8. Return to oven and bake for a further 20-25 minutes at 375.F

I like to make a little tahini, lemon juice, garlic and olive oil sauce to drizzle over the top before eating.

Okinawa, Japan

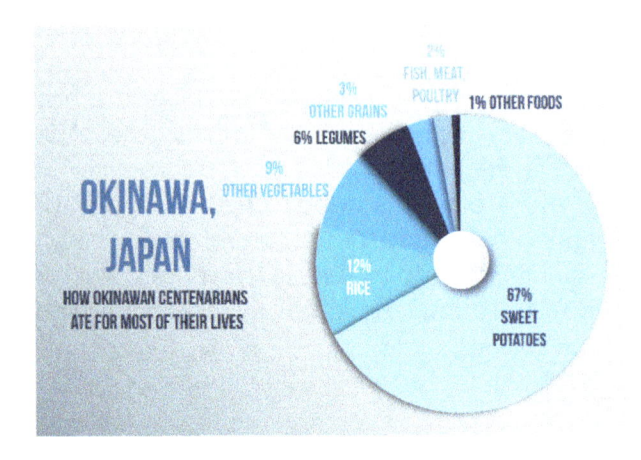

OKINAWA, JAPAN
HOW OKINAWAN CENTENARIANS ATE FOR MOST OF THEIR LIVES

- 67% SWEET POTATOES
- 12% RICE
- 9% OTHER VEGETABLES
- 6% LEGUMES
- 3% OTHER GRAINS
- 2% FISH, MEAT, POULTRY
- 1% OTHER FOODS

The Okinawan Elder's diet primarily consists of 96% vegetables and grains with only 4% of their diet derived from fish, meat or dairy.

Their diet contains these types of vegetables: yams, taro, purple and orange sweet potatoes, seaweed, kelp, bamboo shoots, radish, bitter melon, cabbage, carrots, pumpkin, and mushrooms. They eat a variety of rice. Soba noodles are another staple and are often consumed with broth and vegetables.

The other interesting fact is that the Okinawan's have a rule to stop eating when they are 80% full.

They do eat a small amount of pork, but it is usually reserved for ceremonial occasions or special events.

They enjoy a variety of fruit including citrus fruit, guavas, mangoes, papayas, passion fruit, and pineapples.

They have a wonderful social network for elders called 'moai' which is a group of lifelong friends or a communal structure of people who enjoy the same interests and hobbies.

They have a wonderful saying before eating each meal. They intone three words *'hara hachi bu'*, which translates to 8/10. It translates to 'stop when you are 80% full'. Pretty easy right?

Traditionally, groups of five children were paired together to remain lifelong friends and to support each other throughout life.

Their diet is high in antioxidants. They regularly plant medicinal gardens and enjoy herbs such as ginger, mug wort and turmeric.

Here is an easy delicious Okinawan Soup variation that is vegan, nutritious, and delicious.

Okinawan Udon Noodle Soup

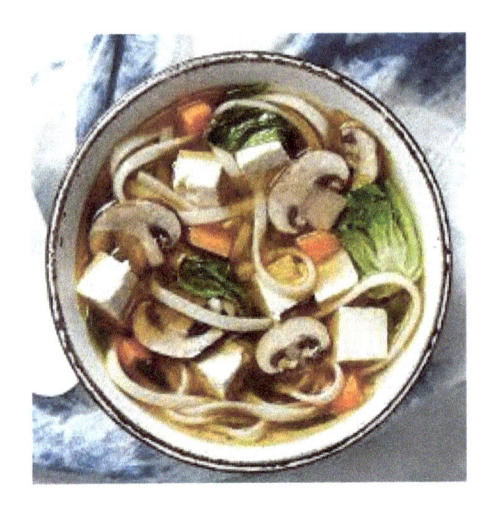

INGREDIENTS

- 1 pack 12 - 14oz Udon Noodles
- 1 package firm tofu, drained and diced
- 4-5 cups of Daishi Umami Broth (which be bought pre-made or as a stock and mixed with boiling water)
- Bok choy or broccoli cut into small bite sized pieces
- ½ cup sliced mushrooms
- ½ cup finely sliced onions
- 5 x scallions/green onions diced
- 1 tablespoon soy sauce
- 1 teaspoon sesame oil (sub olive oil if you don't have it handy)
- 1/3 cup daikon radish cut into small squares
- ¼ cup julienned carrots
- 1 x potato cubed (can be any kind including yam or sweet potato
- 1-2 teaspoons dark sugar to sweeten
- 2 teaspoons grated ginger or 1 teaspoon ginger powder
- Chili flakes (optional)

- Salt and pepper to taste

DIRECTIONS

1. Cook Udon noodles according to the packet
2. Set aside
3. In a large skillet heat oil and add onion. Daikon radish and potato and sauté. Add toku and continue to sauté for 5-6 minutes
4. Pour dashi into skillet and cover. Add all other ingredients (broccoli, carrot, mushrooms, soy sauce & ginger) simmering until all ingredients are tender
5. Taste broth and sweeten or add salt and pepper. Chili flakes optional.
6. Drain and add Udon noodles (cooked separately in step 1)
7. Scoop a portion into a bowl and garnish with green onions, more grated ginger and julienned carrots.

You can add sesame seeds and finely sliced seaweed. This delicious soup keeps in the fridge for several days and it can be enjoyed hot or cold.

Just to recap. What do all of these Blue Zones have in common?

- Sense of community/spend time with friends/engage in social activities

- They eat predominantly fruits, vegetables, and grains

- They exercise regularly

- They eat very little/no dairy

- They eat a very limited amount of meat

- They control their portion sizes/eat until they are 80% full

Not too difficult to do, right? Small changes can make a huge difference to our lives and our wellbeing.

Chapter 13
Diet vs Hereditary

Many doctors now agree that whilst medical conditions can be hereditary, we can change our predispositions through our diet. We are taught so much by our parents. And our parents are taught by their parents.

Many dieticians and medical specialists are starting to see the correlation between the food our parents ate, and passed down to us through recipes and food habits, and a correlation between diseases that appear to run in families.

Take for instance, diabetes. For example, a man in his fifties has just been diagnosed with type 2 diabetes. His father has diabetes and his Grand Mother on his mother's side and his Grand Father on his father's side both died of illnesses which were exacerbated by their diabetes.

The man's diet is rich in meat, potatoes, he loves yoghurt and fruit for breakfast. He eats Mexican food (tacos or burritos) for lunch often. And he loves the beef enchiladas his wife makes. His family loves to BBQ and he frequently entertains cooking BBQ'ed pork chops, steaks and chicken. His wife makes a nice big salad to accompany the meal. And his brother's wife brings her famous macaroni salad. And often a potato salad with lots of mayonnaise. Afterwards they all eat pie and ice cream. He doesn't always indulge but sometimes he just can't resist. It's the weekend. He walks several days during the week and occasionally plays tennis. He golfs with his friends when he can find the time.

Given the history of diabetes in the family one would think that perhaps it is hereditary. No. Not necessarily. Perhaps it is diet. In fact, I know it is his diet.

While it is fine to indulge once in a while, it is not healthy to constantly bombard the body with animal proteins. And it is especially unhealthy when these animal proteins are combined with carbohydrates and refined sugars. *(Remember Chapter 2 on Trophology?)*

Here's why. High cholesterol levels are caused by consuming animal fats and unhealthy oils. If we eat animal products constantly there is so much build up in our systems that we eventually develop hardened arteries leading to heart disease. *And heart disease is the number one cause of death in the majority of western countries.*

The other interesting thing that animal fat does is coat the intestines. Sugar has long been villainized as the cause of diabetes. Contrarily, sugar and carbohydrates are super important fuels for our bodies and brains. The body can absorb sugars through the intestines and convert it to glucose (essential for the brain).

But guess what happens if your stomach and intestines are coated in animal fat? Sugars cannot be absorbed. This leads to an increase in blood sugars and just like that… diabetes. Not to mention the fact that you are also not absorbing many of the important nutrients and minerals of your food through the intestines. If your intestines are coasted in animal fat they simply cannot do their job effectively. It is little wonder that many people in the Western world *actually* suffer from malnutrition.

It would be enough to turn you off animal products, right?

There is also a flip side. Many vegans will disagree vehemently with me on this point, but a small well-proportioned amount of fish or lean meat occasionally is not going to kill you. And this may be different for everyone. For me it means 1-2 times a week I will eat a small 4-6 oz portion of salmon or tuna, sometimes chicken or even grass-fed organic beef. But that's it. That's my limit. Once you become in tune with your body you will find that your body will be the indicator of what you require.

I feel far better and I find I have more energy eating predominantly plant-based, but if I am craving a steak – I eat it. And I enjoy it.

Receiving all of the protein we require by eating plant-based is not always easy and that is why I supplement my diet with a small number of fish or meat.

It is important to note here, that when I do eat lean animal protein it is always accompanied by green vegetables or a large green salad and I even sometimes add some mushrooms or ¼ cup mashed sweet potato.

But What about eating out?

Here's the good news. You don't have to give up eating the foods you love entirely. It's all about finding a balance.

I love schnitzel. Am I going to eat it every day? No. Am I going to eat it occasionally? Yes! To be fair, I haven't eaten schnitzel for over a year. But I do enjoy it.

It's all about finding a healthy balance. For you, that could mean 50% plant based and 50% the foods that contain animal proteins. Bear in mind if you are going to eat these foods, apply the rules of Trophology/food combining to ensure fast, effective digestion. This will ensure that you process these foods quickly and efficiently.

I have found that if I eat 80% plant based and 20% food, I adore but may not necessarily be good for me, and I apply the rules of Trophology, I am able to maintain my weight and even lose weight. I also feel better about what I am putting into my body because I understand that I am allowing my body to digest efficiently and effectively. And yes, I feel better because I am helping the environment too.

I will still always love fine dining and the occasion juicy steak, but I also understand that my body responds better to plant based foods. Once I found a few diet hacks to create ingredients that I was used to cooking with, and replaced them with plant-based alternatives, my dietary confusion was eradicated.

It became easier to understand which foods to eat together and which foods to avoid. I can honestly say that I never feel deprived of any particular food. I just worked out how best to incorporate them into my diet. *And in which order.*

Once the mystery around digestion and efficiently fueling the body becomes clear, your dietary choices open up and you are free to choose.

It is that easy. I promise.

THE SNEAKY AF* DIET BOOK

Chapter 14
But Animals are Tasty
or
Don't Eat The Homies!

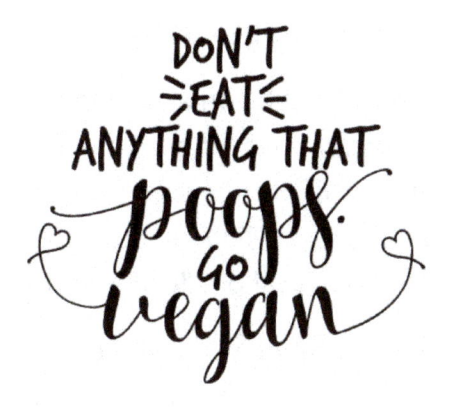

Don't eat anything that poops. Go vegan

I know! And most of the recipes we grew up with contained animal protein, right? Milk, cream, cheese, lard, some even called for suet?! I promise! Check out any traditional English Christmas Pudding recipe. It calls for suet. Some disgusting, cholesterol laden, mixture of animal innards.

If you are reading this in a country that was not once desiccated, raped or pillaged under the guise of the British Empire then this probably reads obsolete for you. But nonetheless, I promise it is true. Google it!

When you consume excessive amounts of cholesterol, in the form of animal fat, you are blocking your arteries. You are causing early onset dementia, heart disease, cancer and the like.

Gone are the days *(my 1990's encounter with eating vegan)* of having to eat pasta with marinara sauce at a restaurant because it is the only plant-based choice! That, or tequila (vegan). Most restaurants now will have many plant-based options or will at least be able to substitute meat with a plant friendly alternative.

I recently flew to Australia to spend time with my family post covid. I had not seen them for 4 whole years. I usually would travel to see them every 12-18 months.

I was particularly impressed by an article in an inflight magazine about a Michelin starred chef who was going to open a steak restaurant but decided to open a vegan restaurant instead. Just to see if he could still get a Michelin star. He's not vegan. He's just about sustainability. Local produce and the like.

He got the Michelin star anyway, all while cooking a completely plant-based menu and I seriously (probably) said out loud 'FUCK YEAH'.

Way to go, dude!

High five!

Way to show them that you are an awesome chef.

But he's not the only one! The world's 'best' restaurant – *Eleven Madison Park*, located in New York, changed its menu to entirely plant-based in 2021.

A Michelin 3-star restaurant choosing to entirely change their menu was a shock to the restaurant world. But he did it! And he still excelled.

Geranium, the Michelin 3 starred restaurant located in Denmark, also announced in 2021 that they would be dropping meat from their menu entirely.

It has never been easier to dine out on enjoyable vegan food. There is a plethora of wonderful plant-based restaurants popping up all over the place.

My local favorite is *Seabirds*. Every time I dine there I am blown away by how delicious the food is. I leave feeling light and energized. Their ingredients are fresh and amazing. I do not miss meat or dairy for a second.

Plant based food can actually taste every bit as amazing as its animal-based rivals without trying to clog our arteries with cholesterol and kill us prematurely.

What a concept. Fine dining using plant-based ingredients. Fine dining, every bit as delicious, 100% better for you. And the great news… you can find every iteration of every recipe using plant-based alternatives. Just google your favorite recipe and add 'vegan' to the end and you will find so many easy to make alternatives.

A smart person once said to me….

MODERATION

IS

THE

THE SNEAKY AF* DIET BOOK

KEY

That's why I called it The Sneaky AF* Diet Book, right? Because it is sneaky in a way that you can begin to harmonize with our own body and seek a truly nourishing diet. All without giving up the things you love.

It's all about balance.

I think I will always enjoy a steak on the BBQ every now and then. Who wouldn't? I'd also like to dispel the popular myth about Australians *(in case you haven't been paying attention – I am an Australian)*.

We do not put shrimp on the barbie (BBQ).

We put steak on the BBQ! And sausages, and chicken, and fish, but never shrimp *(they get a bit dry on the barbie to be quite frank)*.

Once you become harmonized to when your body specifically cries out 'I need a steak" and when you are you just going through the motions of eating what's available in front of you, you will truly be able to discern the difference. I get it.. choosing plant-based options can be tricky when you are under time constraints. It does take a bit more planning to ensure you make good choices.

Hopefully, *if I've done my job right,* you will be able to say – "I'll choose plant based for this meal". And you will feel better. You will look better. You will sleep better. And this will keep you on the path of eating healthy plant friendly foods.

You will also be able to say, "I am looking forward to going out for dinner with my wife/friends/family on Saturday night and I will savor that delicious piece of salmon or chicken parmigiana". Because you know you have been eating right all week and you are adhering to the rule of 80/20.

And hopefully you will only eat until you are 80% full. You will enjoy the dinner with greens and healthy sides and you will pass on the bread basket and the dessert! But hey, Rome wasn't built in a day.

Chapter 15
Choose Alternatives

When I decided to start out on my plant-based journey, I decided on eating vegan for at least 50% of all meals. I realized there were a few recipes that I just loved and never wanted to give up eating. And yes, they contained all the yummy things. Bacon, eggs, cream, cheese.

So, instead of depriving myself I set about making these recipes in a plant-based way. There are loads of recipes on the internet. There are vegan forums on social media.

With a little tweaking, you can still enjoy all your favorite foods.

I know it can seem daunting to cook, and at first, I thought I would have to spend extra hours in the kitchen doing meal preparation.

Then I started to scour the grocery store freezer meals looking for healthy, vegan pre-made frozen meals. I was working 8-9 hours a day and I rarely had time to take a full lunch break, so these microwave ready meals really came in handy.

THE SNEAKY AF* DIET BOOK

I found as long as I made a substantial breakfast and still incorporated lots of fruit and nuts into my diet as snacks I could eat as much as I wanted and never count calories again!

Freedom at last! Not feeling hungry. Not worrying about following a meat-based meal with a dessert. These rules do not apply to vegan eating. You can eat all the plant protein you like and still follow up with a delicious dessert. *I do not recommend doing this all the time,* but it's nice to splurge every now and then.

Remember our chapter on Trophology? Well, when eating plant-based protein our digestive environment remains alkaline meaning we can add carbohydrates and the odd sugary dessert. Who doesn't love dessert?

There are so many cream and ice cream alternatives now that you will never feel deprived.

Here's one dish I knew I could never live without. So, I adapted it to be plant-based and I think it is more delicious than its predecessor. And now I eat this pasta without feeling full and sleepy afterwards! I have made it for many people and everyone loves it.

I am not an advocate for eating simple carbohydrates like pasta every day, but sometimes you've got to live, right?

I hope you enjoy it as much as I do!

Sarah's Favorite Carbonara

(Feeds 4 people)

Ingredients:

- Vegan Pasta (I use Vons Signature Gluten Free as it only contains Rice Flour, Corn Flour)
- Benevolent Bacon. If you cannot find a bacon alternative, you could use vegan sausage sliced and cut into strips
- Half a large brown onion finely chopped
- 2 large chopped garlic cloves or a teaspoon of minced garlic
- 1 cup of frozen Peas (I use petite pois as they are smaller)
- Cashew Cream (I use 1 cup of raw cashews, unsalted) blended with water
- Lots of freshly ground black pepper
- ½ teaspoon of red pepper flakes (optional)
- Nutritional Yeast – It's a cheese replacement (optional)

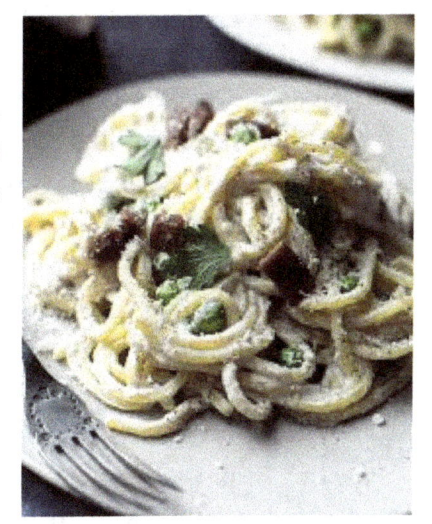

Directions:

1. Finely dice the onion.
2. Soak the cashews in boiling water for 15-25 minutes. Drain and add them to a blender or food processor. Add 1 ½ cups of water and blend. You may need to add more water. You need a consistency a little thicker than heavy cream.
3. Take a large skillet or frying pan. Add a little olive oil and fry up the onions for around 15 minutes on low – medium heat until

soft and translucent. Add the benevolent bacon cut into strips or the vegan sausage. Add the garlic. Turn off the heat and cover until the pasta is ready.
4. Boil a large pot of water. Once it is boiling, add 1 teaspoon and 1 teaspoon of olive oil to prevent the pasta from sticking. Add the pasta. One whole packet of pasta will serve 4 people. For 2 people halve the ingredients or make for 4 people so you have yummy leftovers that will last for 3-4 days in the fridge.
5. Add pasta, stirring often to reduce sticking. I run a fork through the pasta while it is cooking and shake gently. Add the peas and cover the pan so it comes back to a boil.

Once the pasta is ready, drain and return to the large saucepan. Add the onion/bacon/garlic mixture. Add plenty of freshly ground black pepper. Pour the cashew cream over the pasta. Turn the heat onto low and cover for a couple of minutes, stirring well to ensure the pasta is coated in the sauce, and the mixture is incorporated. You may need to add a little more water depending on the consistency of the sauce.

Serve hot with a sprinkle of nutritional yeast or vegan parmesan cheese. I can hardly tell the difference between Trader Joes nondairy parmesan and Italian grated parmesan, especially when added to pasta.

Great Plant-Based Alternatives for Cooking

Butter

There are a lot of fabulous butter alternatives that taste just the same (in my opinion). I usually buy Earth Balance. You can make your own butter!

Here's an easy recipe:

Ingredients:

- ½ cup almond milk
- 1 teaspoon lemon juice
- 1 teaspoon sea salt
- 1 cup oil (canola or olive oil)
- 2 teaspoons liquid aminos or soy sauce
- 4oz cocoa butter
- ½ teaspoon xantham gum
- Either nutritional yeast or a dash of curcumin for color (optional)

Melt the cocoa butter in microwave. Mix all ingredients or blend with an immersion blender.

Put in a Tupperware container with a lid. Refrigerate overnight.

Cream

One cup of blended silken tofu makes a fabulous cream alternative when needed in a recipe. You can add a packet of ranch dressing to one cup of silken tofu for a delicious ranch dressing.

You can also use 1 cup of almond or oat milk with 2 teaspoons of cornstarch as a cream alternative.

Coconut milk is another wonderful substitute.

My favorite is a handful of raw cashews blended with 1 ½ cups filtered water. It has a richer, slightly sweeter taste and it's amazing in cream-based sauces and chowders.

Add some nutritional yeast and a few tablespoons of salsa to your cashew cheese and blend. You now have a delicious queso dip of cheese sauce to add to tacos.

Eggs

Aquafaba (the juice from a can of chickpeas) whips up almost as well as egg whites.

You can sub a banana for eggs in a recipe. They work really well in vegan pancakes.

Apple sauce is another great egg alternative.

One tablespoon of ground flaxseeds or chia seeds combined with three tablespoons of hot water works well as an egg replacement in baked goods.

There are a number of commercial egg replacements, but they can be expensive.

Cheese

Cashew Cheese is very easy to make and it's absolutely delicious.

There are a number of recipes for sweet potato nacho cheese. With the addition of nutritional yeast, it tastes really good. It makes great mac and cheese.

Missing Parmesan cheese? Mix 1 cup of almond flour with 1 teaspoon of garlic powder, 1 teaspoon of onion powder, a little salt, and some nutritional yeast.

A site called thehiddenveggies.com has a number of wonderful, easy-to-make vegan cheese recipes that look exactly like cheese. Add some garlic and herbs to make a delicious creamy cheese alternative.

There are also a number of store-bought alternatives, but they can get expensive!

Meat Alternatives

Mushrooms are a great option in place of meat in recipes. Portobello mushrooms are a great alternative in burgers, and they can be made to taste quite meat-like with the addition of steak seasoning and liquid smoke.

The addition of finely diced mushrooms and cooked brown lentils can be added to stews, casseroles and pasta sauces to replace ground beef.

Tempe is made from fermented soybeans and is molded into a block. It is a wonderful meat alternative due to its texture. It's high in protein and provides around 20 grams per serving.

Tofu can be marinated or crumbled and cooked to add to dishes. Tofu is wonderfully versatile and as it has a mild taste it is a great candidate for marinades and spices.

Jackfruit is a great meat alternative due to its fleshy texture. It makes a wonderful pulled 'pork' with the addition of BBQ sauce.

It's high in vitamins A, B & C. Unfortunately, it is not high in protein, but the addition of lentils or chickpeas will ensure adequate protein.

Walnuts and pecans can be finely chopped and added in place of meat. They are naturally high in protein and the fat in nuts is slowly absorbed by the body making it preferable over meat.

Nuts contain plant sterols which help keep cholesterol levels in check and reduce the risk of cancer.

Seitan is another less common meat alternative. There are several recipes that turn seitan into a beef pot roast.

It is high in protein and low in carbohydrates and fat. It contains a high amount of iron and selenium making it a great choice if you are looking to add protein to your diet.

Chapter 16
Isn't Eating Plant Based Expensive?

There is a super easy answer to this question! If you choose processed, vegan alternatives, then YES! It can get very expensive!

Fortunately, there are alternatives.

Take for instance, the impossible burger.

A burger patty is going to run you $2 - $3 if you buy at a store in a 6 pack, whereas a burger patty will cost you around $0.75 - $1.00.

Choose a vegie burger patty instead? They will run you around $0.50 - $0.75 when purchased in a multi-pack. And many contain more protein than a beef burger or an impossible burger patty. *I always opt for ones that contain lentils or beans which are a wonderful clean source of protein.*

The great news is that the vegie burger option will contain far less saturated fat making it a healthier option.

How about a spaghetti Bolognese sauce? A package of organic, grass-fed ground beef will run you $8 - $9. Sub this for precooked brown lentils and finely chopped mushrooms and you will save around $4 and easily feed 4 people for around $12 - $15.

The price of eggs has skyrocketed (at the time of writing this). You will pay around $6 - $8 for organic free-range eggs whereas a tofu alternative will cost you around $1.69. Ever tried scrambled tofu? Spice it up and it's actually rather delicious!

Egg alternatives can be expensive ($5.99 per container) so improvise! I love lentils on toast. And beans on toast. These are both high protein alternatives which are cheap and easy to prepare quickly. And the great news! No cholesterol.

I will still occasionally eat eggs, but they are definitely not part of my daily diet any longer.

Looking for an egg alternative to add to a recipe? Try Aquafaba. *(Don't worry – it's a fancy word for bean juice).*

When you empty a can of chickpeas or beans, reserve the juice. It has a similar texture to egg whites and whips up nearly as well.

There are so many delicious, nutritious pancake recipes online that use a mashed banana instead of an egg! This way you are receiving good healthy carbs, potassium, magnesium, B6 and a healthy source of sugar.

Jackfruit is a fleshy fruit native to Southeast Asia. It is a wonderful meat alternative. Seasoned just right and added to a taco I find it better than meat. Dress it up with BBQ sauce and add a little slaw – bam! You have a delicious and nutritious pulled jackfruit slider. It's high in protein, Vitamins B & C, and potassium. Due to its recent popularity, it is readily available canned or fresh-frozen. It's inexpensive too. Trader Joes even have a BBQ jackfruit ready to heat and add to a salad or a bun.

Mushrooms are a fabulous alternative to meat. A cooked and seasoned portobello mushroom burger is delicious and very inexpensive to make. They are naturally low in carbohydrates and high in fiber.

Craving a hot dog? There are a multitude of vegan sausages and hot dogs available that are delicious. And you skip all of the animal fat and cholesterol associated with a regular hot dog.

I know I am listing rather unhealthy foods above, but these are often fast go-to options for people. There is a plethora of healthy options without including complex carbohydrates like bread and pasta.

Vegan meals do work out less expensive when averaged out so long as you are incorporating great alternatives like rice, beans, lentils, nuts, oats, flaxseed, quinoa and whole grains.

Chapter 17
Fasting/Cleanses

We are what we eat! Most of us have been trained to eat several meals a day with snacks in between meals.

We have been taught to exercise more and eat less. As we age, excessive cardio exercise can lead to mTor activation. What we can physically handle when we are younger, often no longer suits us as we age.

Overeating taxes the pancreas and digestive system. Eating late at night can lead to digestive issues. Our body does not have the necessary time to digest our food effectively before we go to bed.

Here's where restricting our eating to a specific time window can be effective. It's called intermittent fasting and it can be a great tool for weight loss.

We have become consumers in the Western world. Many Americans work in jobs where they are sedentary for a large portion of the day. They not only eat 3 meals a day, but they snack in between.

THE SNEAKY AF* DIET BOOK

It is crucial to give our bodies a break from digestion. One of the single most detrimental things we can do for our health is to eat late at night before going to sleep.

Fasting is a super important part of the wellness equation. It has been somewhat of a buzz word lately. Intermittent fasting, juice cleanses, water fasting… the list goes on.

Fasting need not be so extreme though.

Many people should not fast due to medical conditions.

I learned about this simple and highly effective 'cleanse' that can be as good as fasting.

It's super easy and you can still eat exactly the way you would normally eat. You just need to add in a couple of products to your daily routine.

EASY CLEANSE

1. Bentonite – I recommend Sonnes brand for its purity and quality.
2. Psyllium Husk – I always buy the Gluten Free variety.

When you wake up mix 1 tablespoon of bentonite with 1 tablespoon of psyllium husk in an 8 oz glass of water. Drink immediately. Wait 45 minutes – 1 hour before consuming food.

Eat your normal diet during the day. Try to finish eating by 7pm. Before you go to bed, consume 1 tablespoon of bentonite with 1 tablespoon of psyllium husk in 8oz glass of water. Do not eat anything after this.

Repeat this process for 4-6 weeks.

The great thing about bentonite (volcanic ash) is that it can carry 1,000 times its molecular weight of junk and toxins from the intestines.

One of my friends lost 15 pounds from just doing this cleanse for 6 weeks. She was struggling with her weight, and she came to me for advice, I recommended the above and within 6 weeks she had lost a substantial amount of weight and felt great. She now routinely factors this cleanse into her wellness regime and completes the above every 6 months.

ADOPTING A 14/10 BALANCE

This is pretty much my comfort point. I like to eat at 9 am every day. I have a light breakfast. I have my last meal around 6:30 pm and I do not eat anything after 7 pm.

I eat for 10 hours. I fast for 14 hours. You can adapt this in any way that works best with your schedule. Perhaps you like to eat at 8 am. Then you would have your last meal around 5:30 pm.

Perhaps you are not hungry until lunch. Eat your first meal at noon. Finish your last meal by 10 pm, however, do not go to bed immediately following your last meal. Wait a few hours.

Another useful tip is to do a little light exercise after a big meal. It could be a 10–15-minute walk around your neighborhood. It could be a quick trip to the gym. It could be a 15-minute mat yoga class. Whatever it is, it does help the digestive process if we do some form of exercise after a meal.

The first 2 weeks of adopting this 14/10 dietary rule were absolute hell. I went to bed every night. My stomach was rumbling. I didn't sleep properly. I had *(fortunately)* watched a few YouTube videos on Intermittent Fasting. This had prepared me for a little sleeplessness and discomfort initially.

I just had to push through it, and once I did, I was astounded by how much better I felt. I no longer awoke starving hungry. In fact, I woke up feeling great. I was no longer hungry in the evenings. Even if I went out and had a few drinks. Usually, I'd arrive home and eat a late-night snack. I'd tell myself it would help absorb the alcohol and reduce a hangover. Negative. In fact, it does the opposite. If you've overloaded your system with alcohol, the last thing you want to do is overload it even more by having to digest food.

For some people the rule of 16/8 works – they eat for 8 hours and fast for 16 hours.

Find a healthy happy balance. And remember the more you switch your diet to plant based – the less hungry you will be. This is a fascinating and wonderful fact. I always thought I had some kind of blood sugar issue as I was hungry every 4 hours. Now I only eat when I'm hungry. The more plant-based my diet is, the less hungry I am. And your taste buds do actually change. It takes a while but you will start to find you crave healthy foods instead of salty sugary ones.

Juice Fasting

Extreme juice fasts should only be done under medical supervision. They can be highly effective. There are numerous stories of people curing serious illnesses and ailments by going on a juice fast.

But again, doctor supervision is recommended especially if you are suffering from a serious illness. There are many wonderful retreats around the world that offer juice fasts with medical doctors to monitor your progress.

Chapter 18
The 8 Limbs of Yoga (The Roadmap to Happiness)

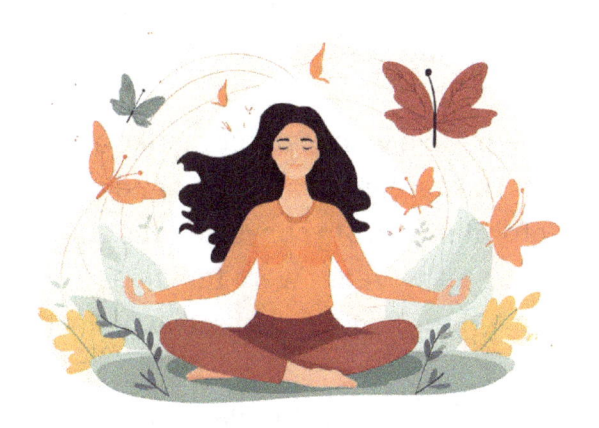

The reason I am addressing yoga is this chapter is purely to draw light to the essence of the original teachings. When we think of yoga, we think of the exercises (Asana), that have been adopted in the west. In a sense, we have culturally appropriated a small part of yoga and rebranded the exercise portion as 'yoga'. Many of us do not truly understand the heart of the teachings and it is this portion or 'whole' that I would like to delve into.

Here is an interesting theory I learned from one of my yoga teachers. She was my teacher on my month-long yoga teacher training sabbatical in Thailand. It goes something like this...

THE SNEAKY AF* DIET BOOK

The yogic Vedas were taught widely in India over 5,000 years ago. This was before people had the ability to read and write. Many of the villagers were simple farm workers. The yogic Vedas were taught in a way to encompass all three methods of learning:

1. Kinesthetic - Through movement – the type of yoga we have come to know today in the west. This is particularly important as people who are kinesthetic learners learn primarily through movement. They often become chiropractors, massage therapists, dancers and the like.

2. Auditory – people who learn primarily via audio methods. They are great at listening to lectures and retain information from conversations and from the spoken word. The Vedas were taught as a chant which accompanied the sequence of movements (Asana).

3. Visual – people who learn visually do great when there is a slideshow. They can follow along by learning and observing visually, and this is reinforced via audio (often in the form of a teacher talking or lecturer). They can often be found staring blankly out a window during a lecture that has no visual component. People who learn visually often have photographic memories. The Vedas were taught by observing and following the Yogis performing the sequence of movements.

The yogis travelled extensively through India. They went from village to village teaching the yogic Vedas. This way, the Vedas were handed down to lay people who often could not read and write.

The yogis understood the importance of being able to reinforce the Vedas by teaching them in the three ways mentioned above. The Vedas were taught and displayed by movement. Disciples could copy the range of movements by observing visually, chanting the Vedas (audio) and practicing the accompanying movements. Thus, they could learn to commit the Vedas to heart and incorporate them into their lives.

Most people are a makeup of both audio/visual. Visual learners usually have a harder time in a classroom where many of the lessons are delivered via audio methods. Good teachers understand the necessity to present some form of visual context along with the audio. The yogis understood, even back then, that reinforcing their teaching with all 3 methods could garner faster learning and retention.

So, why do the 8 limbs of yoga factor in?

In short, because they are a roadmap by which to live a happier, more fulfilling life.

Yoga is much more than having a great limber body with toned abdominal muscles. In fact, the exercises are only one small part of yoga as a whole. Yoga was designed to be a spiritual pathway, not a path to a flat belly. And while I highly recommend the practice of yogic exercise, I would like to also discuss the positivity of embracing The Eight Limbs of Yoga.

The 8 Limbs of Yoga

THE SNEAKY AF* DIET BOOK

1. YAMAS
   There are 5 Yamas:

   - AHIMSA – Nonviolence, treating all sentient beings with respect and love. This also includes extending this love, respect and kindness to ourselves. It also includes practicing kindness to animals *(and not eating them!)*.

   - SATYA – Truthfulness, of the spoken word. Doing our best to maintain integrity and honesty in all of our dealings with others. If truth may hurt another, often silence is our best option.

   - BRAHMACHARYA – Fidelity, doing our best to honor and respect our friends and even showing kindness to those who wrong us. Using our best intentions and efforts to be our best selves.

   - APARIGRAHA – Non-Greed – Understanding we are already enough. Also, when we find ourselves fortunate enough to have more than we need – using our resources to help others. A simple act of kindness of helping another being or giving up something we no longer need to someone less fortunate, is of great importance.

2. NIYAMAS
   There are 5 Niyamas

- SAUCHA - Cleanliness – this is so important in the disposable world we live in today. This doesn't just mean to clean your house; it means to keep the planet clean. Recycle. Buy less plastic. Compost. Create less waste. To keep not only the space immediately surrounding us tidy, but to make an effort to keep this beautiful world healthy.

- SANTOSHA – Happiness/Contentment – not just our own personal happiness but the happiness of those around us too. Appreciating what we have and taking time to reflect on this beautiful planet we are lucky enough to live on.

- SVADHYAYA – Learning from Mistakes/Humility – this includes admitting our part in conflicts and problems and not being afraid to say I am sorry. Letting go of ego and the need to be right. Allowing ourselves to move forwards, away from the past and towards the future. Understanding it is ok to forgive others and to forgive ourselves.

- Ishvara Pranidhana – Having Faith – this can mean having faith in whatever you believe in. It could be God. It could be Buddha. It could be your dog. Or it could be Mother Nature (Aya). Whatever your beliefs, it is a wonderful feeling to surrender to the divine. To know everything will be ok, if we just keep the faith.

THE SNEAKY AF* DIET BOOK

3. ASANA – In the tradition yoga sense, asana relates to a series of movement that were traditionally taught with chants (yogic Vedas). Yoga asana today has been broadly adopted by the west including classes that can be extremely challenging like Ashtanga or more restorative in nature like Iyengar.

   But let's look at asana in a completely different way. Let's view asana as any kind of movement or exercise that you enjoy. It could be walking the dog in the park, a competitive game of pickleball, martial arts, swimming, hiking, golfing, surfing…. The list goes on.

   But what is really important, is committing to doing some kind of exercise each and every day. The yogis liked to do their sun salutations in the morning. There is a very good reason for this. During the night we accumulate toxins. Our body slows down, our digestion decreases, and our bodies engage in a constant restorative/repair cycle that only happens best when we are asleep. Our body is always working to remove toxins from the body whether they are airborne, from the food we have consumed or from the stress of our everyday lives.

   As a result, when we get up and move in the morning, our lymphatic system needs to be stimulated. This allows the stored toxins to circulate and be released through the breath. Moving allows our bodies to expel this waste built up efficiently and effectively. This lymphatic circulation is imperative to our wellbeing.

Ever wondered why there is an emergence of heart disease, lymphatic cancers, strokes and the like? We are designed to move. Yet a good portion of our lives are spent stationary. We sit at an office desk. We binge watch Netflix. We sat and watched a movie. Follow this up with a diet high in animal fat and the results are disastrous.

Even if you can only assign 10-15 minutes in the morning to stretch and move – Do It! I cannot stress the importance of this enough.

4. PRANAYAMA – and this is where the ancient practice of pranayama comes into play. Quite literally, it means to control the flow of energy within the body. The lifeforce.

   It could be accomplished through silent meditation and focus on the breath. It could be accomplished by dedicating time every day to a series of life changing yogic breathing exercises (I will outline a few at the end of this chapter).

   It could be accomplished by lifting weights and focusing on inhaling the breathe in, lifting the weight, and exhaling the breath out, releasing the weight. There is no right or wrong. One thing the yogis did understand is that to breathe is to circulate prana (energy) throughout the body.

Often in a yoga class the teacher will draw attention to the breath. Students beginning to practice yoga can have a habit of holding their breath and stilting the prana within the body.

Pranayama breathing exercise can take years to master, and they can be very powerful. The ones outlined later in this chapter are quite simple and do not take a huge amount of time. In fact, they can be practiced anywhere.

5. PRATYAHARA – This is the practice of detaching from external and surrounding distractions and drawing the awareness back into the body. It can be done whilst walking in the park (preferably without headphones!). It can be done waiting in the queue at the grocery store.

    It is all about tapping into the inner peace that exists in the core of our hearts. Finding that moment of peace and joy even when the world around us is chaotic.

    Maybe you find your true pratyahara while surfing a wave or climbing a rockface. Maybe you find it in the quiet hours of your home before anyone else is awake.

    Wherever you find it, once you begin to tap into this majestic and mystical sense of self, your life will change for the better. I promise you.

Our intuition is a sense that is often overlooked in the west. It can be our guiding beacon and our savior. We just need to place this trust and focus to look within. Everything we need is right inside of ourselves.

6. DHARANA – the practice of intense concentration and focus. Again, this can be achieved wherever you find your peace. It could be cooking a delicious plant-based meal for your family. It could be a task at work that you enjoy. It could be a candlelight meditation. Or a walk on the beach.

   This can be viewed as training the brain to be still. In the world today, we are bombarded with information, some of it useful and some of it useless. From social media to work emails, texts, advertisements, the list goes on and on. It is important to take a break away from this barrage of sensory overload and to just find focus and concentration on a single task.

   And it does not necessarily have to be practiced alone. Maybe you and your partner decide to engage in a loving practice of dharana, sitting quietly in front of each other, eyes closed, palms touching. Focusing on good intentions for each other and those around you.

7. DHYANA – the state of acute awareness letting go of judgement. Let's face it, life today can make it easy to be judgmental of others. I strongly believe social media

plays a large role in this.

But when we let go of judgement of others (and of ourselves) we start to realize that everyone is going through something that we cannot entirely understand. Keeping focus and releasing judgment allows us to become our best selves. It also allows us to relate to others in a more compassionate way.

Dhyana can often be referred to as 'being in the flow'. Athletes often tap into this state. Nothing around them matters. They lose sense of time, sound, and distractions. They enter a state of complete focus.

The Silva method is a wonderful teaching course that outlines how to enter the states of Alpha, Theta and Beta quickly and effectively.

8. SAMADHI – This is referred to often in Buddhist terms as 'enlightenment'. It is a state of bliss. And while it is not possible to live our entire lives in Samadhi *(unfortunately)*, it is most certainly possible to enjoy glimpses and even prolonged periods of Samadhi.

    Tapping into your purpose, your God-given right, can provide a profound sense of Samadhi. This can be a difficult prospect when we have families to look after and financial commitments. I get it, most of us have to work a job which may not fit our ideal, fulfilling purpose. Even if you a have busy schedule, you may find your

Samadhi by volunteering at a local food collective, joining a hiking club, volunteering at an aquarium, playing volleyball, joining a cycling club, taking a gym class or a meditation class or even finding a beekeeping group. It could be learning to paint or taking a few hours on the weekend to capture wildlife photos.

Whatever it is – commit to finding what truly makes your soul sing. Don't ever be afraid to try new things. You are never too old. In fact, this can be the one thing that keeps us young. Be a forever student of life.

As you can see the 8 limbs of yoga are more than just exercises. They are simple practical solutions that we can put to work in our everyday lives without too much extraneous effort.

As a side note, the 8 Limbs of Yoga are very similar to the Eightfold Path of Buddhism. But as I wanted to keep this book as religiously non-denominational as possible, I have chosen the 8 Limbs of Yoga. For those wanting to seek out the Buddhist Eightfold Path, there are many wonderful books and texts available.

Below are some Pranayama Exercises – Some simple and effective breathing routines to circulate and control the flow of energy within the body.

Pranayama Breathing Exercises

ANILOMA VILOMA

(Alternate nostril breathing)

This practice should ideally be done in a seated position. A quiet location is a plus. I like to practice pranayama sitting cross-legged, on my yoga mat, sitting on the edge of a bolster or cushion to move my knees closer to the floor. It can be practiced sitting in a chair or even propped up in bed or leaning against a wall for extra back support.

Instructions for Aniloma Viloma:

- Softly close your eyes and draw attention to the breath.

- Take 4 long, deep inhalations and exhalations through the nostrils.

- Still the mind and draw focus within the body.

- With the thumb of your right hand, gently push against the right nostril, exhaling fully through the left nostril

- Inhale to the count of 4 (1,2,3,4) through your left nostril

- Place your index finger over the left nostril (right thumb is still over the right nostril), and hold your breath for 2 counts (1,2)

- Release your thumb from the right nostril (forefinger is still over the left nostril) and exhale through the right nostril for a count of 4 (1,2,3,4)

- Inhale through the right nostril for a count of 4 (1,2,3,4)

- Place right thumb over right nostril and hold the breath for a count of 2 (1,2)

- Release the forefinger and exhale out of the left nostril

- Always start and end with the left nostril.

Repeat this process for several rounds. Pause and sit quietly allowing the breathing to return normal.

As you get more acquainted with this process of Aniloma Viloma you can increase the count of inhalation/exhalation to a 6 count or 8 count.

It is always important to start inhaling through the left nostril and finish the round exhaling through the left nostril. There is a wonderful reason for this. The left side of our body consists of moon energy, and the right-side sun energy. A perfect balance. In times of stress or excitement you may find that you are breathing predominantly through your right nostril.

Ever noticed it is easier to fall asleep on your right side – predominantly breathing through the left nostril?

Aniloma Viloma allows us to balance this energy or 'prana' or 'chi'.

It is a particularly useful tool in times of stress or anxiety.

It is a balancing breathing technique.

UJJAYI BREATHING

(For focus and concentration)

This particular kind of breath work is particularly popular amongst yogis. It draws focus to the breath and can help to extend and go deeper into postures.

It can be adopted for any kind of work out or training session.

Instructions for Ujjayi:

- As you breath in through the nose, restrict the back of the throat

- You can do this by pushing the tongue to the roof of the mouth

- Make the breath slow and deliberate

- Exhale slowly through the nose

Repeat this process.

Ujjayi breath makes a sound like the ocean or a wave. It can sound like the beginning of a snore!

KAPALABHATI BREATHING

Kapalabhati breathing is vigorous and warms the body. It can help you to sleep better and achieve deeper relaxation.

It is best practiced sitting in a cross-legged position on a mat or a cushion (especially when engaging the Bundhas).

It is particularly useful after a large meal as it can aid in digestion. It has been used for centuries in yoga and is believed to dispel toxins from the body.

It is a cleansing sequence of breath work. This breathing exercise can be done with or without the Bandha locks.

Understanding the Bandhas:

The Bandhas are powerful locks which circulate *prana* or energy throughout the body.

These 3 locks are engaged together.

They can leave you feeling energized and full of positivity.

1. Mula Bundha – this is the root lock which engages the root chakra. It is engaged by tightening the pelvic floor muscles without tightening the buttocks.

2. Uddiyana Bundha – this is the sacral lock that is associated with the sacral and solar plexus chakras. It is engaged by scooping the muscles up and under the ribcage. Think of it like a tiny strand of pearls that engage from the pelvic floor all the way to the belly button.

3. Jalandhara Bhanda – This is the 3ʳᵈ root lock and it is engaged by dropping the chin towards the chest while keeping a straight spine.

Instructions for Kapalabhati:

- Inhale deeply through the nostrils filling the belly with air

- Exhale short, forceful breaths through the nostrils until you have no more air to expel.

- Inhale fully through the nostrils.

- Hold the breath

- Engage Mula Bhanda, Uddiyana Bhanda and Julandhara Bundha while retaining the breath.

- Hold the breath for as long and feels comfortable and slowly release the breath through the mouth. Release the Bhanda locks. Sit comfortably with the eyes closed, relaxing the shoulders.

- Allow breath to return to normal for 5-6 breaths.

Repeat this process 2-3 times.

BHASTRIKA

Bhastrika Breathing is similar to Kapalabhati breathing and it is used to increase prana within the body.

It is a great exercise for reducing blood sugar levels and maintaining a healthy weight.

It can often be referred to as the breath of fire.

Instructions for Bhastrika Breathing:

- Sit comfortably

- Take a few normal breaths

- Inhale sharply and deeply through the nose into the abdomen

- Push the breath out quickly through the nose

Repeat this process 10 - 15 times

It is similar to Khapalabhati but it involves sharp inhalations and exhalations.

LION'S BREATH

Lion's breath is a cleansing exercise. It can help to expand the lungs and eliminate toxins from the body.

THE SNEAKY AF* DIET BOOK

It is also very useful to alleviate anxiety and stress.

There is also a yoga pose known as 'roaring lion' where you start sitting on the heels and as you exhale you come up onto all fours like a roaring lion.

Instructions for Lion's Breath:

- Start in a comfortable seated position

- Take a few deep inhalations and exhalations

- Inhale slowly and deeply through the nose

- Exhale fully and deeply with your mouth wide open and your tongue sticking out as far as possible

Repeat this process. You are eliminating toxins from the body!

Chapter 19
The Chakras

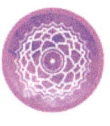

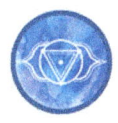

Sahasrara		CROWN CHAKRA
Ajna		THIRD EYE CHAKRA
Visuddha		THROAT CHAKRA
Anahata		HEART CHAKRA
Manipura		SOLAR PLEXUS CHAKRA
Svadhisthana		SACRAL CHAKRA
Muladhara		ROOT CHAKRA

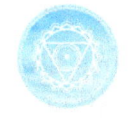

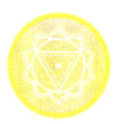

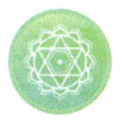

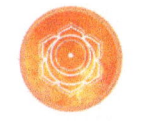

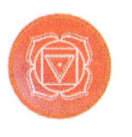

The Chakras are energy centers within the body. The word 'chakra' literally translates to 'wheel' in Sanskrit. The Chakras were first mentioned in the Yogic Vedas which dates back to 1500 BC. The Vedas are believed to be one of the oldest texts.

Chakras were often thought of as an airy, new age term. They link up to several major nerve plexuses and the body's Endocrine System. Eastern medicine has always viewed the energy and flow within the body as a vital component to wellbeing.

Western medicine now views this energy force as a 'biofield'. Integrative medicine takes into consideration lifestyle, body, mind, and energy when diagnosing a patient.

There are many ways to balance chakras and promote the flow of energy within the body, some of which have been provided in this book.

- Mantras

- Pranayama

- Meditation

- Eating a Plant-based diet

- Yoga and exercise

THE CROWN CHAKRA

The Crown Chakra is referred to as 'Sahasrara'. It translates to 'thousands' in Sanskrit and it is often depicted as a lotus flower with a thousand petals.

It is the 7th chakra, and it is directly linked to The Endocrine system which includes the hypothalamus, pineal gland, and the pituitary gland. It is located on the crown of the head.

When the Crown Chakra is balanced you will feel more motivated. You will feel connected to the divine, you will feel an increase in empathy and compassion. You will have a sense of purpose and you will feel connected to all beings. *(So don't eat the homies!)*

Contrarily, when there is a blockage within the Crown Chakra you may feel lost, lacking purpose and disconnected. You may have a sensitivity to light and sound.

Often people will suffer from headaches and insomnia when their Crown Chakra is blocked.

Some affirmations for balancing the Crown Chakra:

- Divinity resides within me
- I am open to new concepts and ideas

- Information I need comes to me easily and helps me to make the right decisions

- The world is my teacher, and I am a willing student

- I am guided by my Higher Power

- I trust my intuition and my inner wisdom

THE THIRD EYE CHAKRA

The Third Eye Chakra is referred to as 'Ajna'. It is the 6th chakra, and it is directly linked to the pineal gland. It is located between the eyebrows and is often depicted a as a third eye.

Ajna is linked to self-awareness, intuition, and a 6th sense. It is linked to a divine knowledge. It is linked to imagination and creativity.

When the Third Eye Chakra is balanced you are able to tune into your intuition and you can make decisions easily and with a sense of positivity. You feel drawn to creating and helping others.

A blockage can lead to anxiety, fogginess, nightmares, and indecision.

Meditation can help to clear the Third Eye Chakra. Closing the eyes and drawing attention to the space between the eyebrows can help to balance this chakra.

Some affirmations for balancing the Third Eye Chakra are:

- I am the source of truth
- My intuition guides me each day
- I am connected to the wisdom of the Universe
- I honor my intuition and allow it to guide me
- I allow good situations and people into my life
- I am aligned with my true purpose
- I am creative and innovative

THE THROAT CHAKRA

The Throat Chakra is referred to as 'Vissuddha'. It is the 5th chakra, and it is directly linked to the thyroid and parathyroid glands.

It is located at the base of the throat. The Throat Chakra is linked to our voice and our ability to speak our truth.

A balanced Throat Chakra will result in a sense of well-being, the ability to communicate clearly, dismissiveness of speech, and authentic expression.

A blocked throat chakra may result in disharmonious relationships, fear of judgement and an inability to communicate.

The sound 'Ohm' is a wonderful clearer of the throat chakra.

Some affirmations for balancing the Throat Chakra are:

- I am the source of truth

- I speak my mind with clarity

- I am happy and comfortable setting clear boundaries

- I trust in my voice and my opinion

- I believe people respect my opinion and straightforwardness

- I am confident

- I am honest and truthful

THE HEART CHAKRA

The Heart Chakra is referred to as 'Anahata'. It translates to 'unhurt' in Sanskrit. It is linked to the heart, the lungs and the thymus gland.

The Heart Chakra is responsible for loving and forgiving. It is the 4th Chakra. People with a healthy balanced heart chakra are loving and kind. They often greet with a hug.

An unbalanced heart chakra can cause one to isolate and feel disconnected. They often do not have a sense of belonging or community.

They can often feel lonely or jealous of others. They often take on the role of 'the victim'.

- I exude Love and Forgiveness
- I am supreme love
- Love surrounds me always
- I love myself and others unconditionally
- I am fulfilling my heart's desire every day
- My heart is free from hurts, past and present
- I choose joy and happiness
- I am open to giving and receiving love

THE SOLAR PLEXUS CHAKRA

The Solar Plexus Chakra is referred to as 'Manipura'. It translates to 'place of the shining gem' in Sanskrit. It is located around 2 inches above the belly button. It is linked to the pancreas and digestive organs.

THE SNEAKY AF* DIET BOOK

The solar plexus chakra is imperative to self-confidence and unlocking your personal power. It also relates to willpower.

It is responsible for effective digestion. The solar plexus manages your fight or flight response. The norepinephrine released by your body when you are stressed redistributes blood away from the digestive organs and to the brain.

This is important as you want effective digestion to stay slim! Limiting stress is key.

An unbalanced solar plexus chakra may result in weight gain due to poor digestion, indigestion, IBS, and ulcers. People who have an imbalance may feel irritable or angry, have low self-confidence, and may seek excessive approval from others.

Some affirmations for balancing the Solar Plexus Chakra are:

- I am ready for any new challenge
- I stand tall in my personal power
- Positive change and harmony flow to me
- I am non-reactive in stressful situations
- I do not need approval from others to know I am complete and perfect
- I pursue my purpose with vigor and happiness
- I create positive change in my life

THE SACRAL CHAKRA

The Sacral Chakra is referred to as 'Svadhisthana'. It translates to 'dwelling place of the self' in Sanskrit. It is located below the belly button, and it is linked to the sex organs.

The Sacral Chakra gives us a sense of confidence in our intimate relationships. It relates to desire and sexual attraction.

A well-balanced Sacral Chakra will ensure you have healthy relationships. It is also connected to our sense of the divine. It is responsible for feeling pleasure.

A blocked Sacral Chakra will often result in lower abdominal pain. People can experience back pain, urinary tract infections, ovarian cysts, and even impotence.

Some affirmations for balancing the Sacral Chakra are:

- I am a passionate person
- I am in control of my emotions
- My passions are fulfilled
- I am not averse to change. I welcome positive changes in my life
- My healthy boundaries protect me

THE SNEAKY AF* DIET BOOK

THE ROOT CHAKRA

The Root Chakra is located at the base of the spine and pelvic floor. It is the 1st Chakra and it is called 'Muladhara' in Sanskrit. Its name translates to 'base or root support'.

The Root Chakra is connected to the bowels and excretory organs. It is responsible for removing toxins from the body.

Muladhara is responsible for our primal sense of survival and grounding. Having a balanced Root Chakra will help you to make instinctive decisions with ease and clarity.

Contrarily, an unbalanced Root Chakra can lead to anxiety, panic attacks, issues with the bowels or colon, fear of financial insecurity, hoarding, and self-pity.

Some affirmations for balancing the Root Chakra are:

- I feel safe and secure in my life
- I am connected to the earth
- I honor Mother Nature
- My roots are strong, just like an oak tree
- I trust the universe and its ability to direct me
- I am getting healthier and stronger every day
- I love myself unconditionally

Chapter 20
Laughter is the best Medicine!

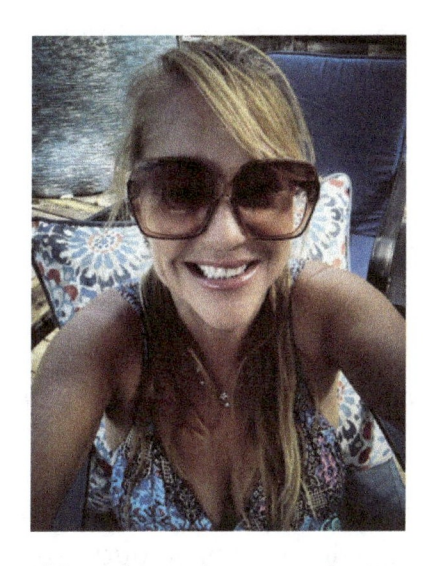

"A smile costs nothing, but gives much. It enriches those who receive it, without making poorer those who give. It takes but a moment, but the memory of it sometimes lasts forever. None is so rich or mighty that he can get along without it, and none is so poor but that he can be made rich by it"
`*Author Unknown*

I remember this saying by heart. My dad had found it in some magazine and posted it on the back of the dunny door (toilet) which it stayed for many years. You couldn't help but read it when going No.2.

Smile more! Smiles are the precursor to laughter. When we smile more – we will definitely laugh more. Try it! Instead of looking down at your phone in the queue at the store, smile at someone. They will usually smile back. Which opens the door to a quick conversation and possibly a laugh!

Laughter and happiness are definitely the keys to an enjoyable life. Sometimes it takes a conscious effort to remain happy and in the moment.

Surround yourself with fun and playful people. Do something silly to make someone laugh. Dance! Remember the child inside and have fun.

Move towards laughter. Have you ever been at an event or a party where somebody is making everyone laugh? Move towards the joy of pure laughter and join in!

Fortunately, there are many tools at our disposal to become happier, healthier individuals. I have outlined a few in this book but it is by no means the only way.

Here are some benefits of laughing:

- Laughter burns calories! Honestly! Laughing 10 minutes per day burns around 50 calories. What a great way to lose weight.

- Laughter improves your immune system. Laughter decreases stress hormones and increases the production of immunity cells.

- Laughter combats stress and anxiety. It helps to relax muscles for up to 45 minutes after a good 'laughter session'.

- Laughter increases blood flow throughout the body bringing fresh blood and circulation to the internal organs and providing the skin with a healthy glow.

- Laughter triggers the release of good endorphins that help you feel good – not just in the moment but for hours to come.

Once you realize you have tools to deal with stress, anxiety or just the plain old blues, you understand how to shift out of the negative and into the positive.

A walk on the beach with my dog always shifts my focus. As does restorative yoga. Even 5 minutes of pranayama (breathing exercises) at my desk will help change my perception.

10-15 minutes watching a comedian on Netflix or watching a feel-good podcast on YouTube will help me to change mode. Distractions can be good.

Not every day is going to be perfect. We all have challenges we will face. It's rather more about how we react. Sometimes stepping away from a situation briefly or taking a moment to meditate on the situation will help to tap into the correct response.

And sometimes when something goes wrong, we can choose to see the pure comedy in the situation. I am not talking about making light of serious situations. Don't berate yourself for small things that go awry. Try to see the humor in each situation.

Learn, grow and share. Life is meant to be shared and savored.

Chapter 21
The Gratitude Jar

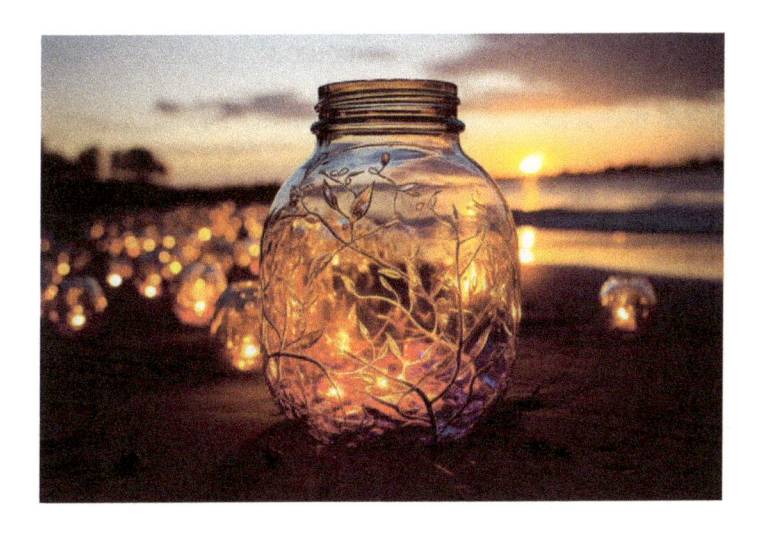

"We can complain because rose bushes have thorns, or we can rejoice because thorn bushes have roses"
~ Abraham Lincoln

Expressing gratitude is so important. We live in an age of social media. It can be easy to slip into a state of dissolution as we see photos of people looking amazing and having fun. It can be hard not to compare our lives to those of airbrushed, photoshopped celebrities.

THE SNEAKY AF* DIET BOOK

We can lose track of what we ought to be grateful for. Each and every one of us have hundreds if not thousands of things to be grateful for every single day.

Starting a Gratitude Jar can be a wonderful way to remind ourselves of our daily blessings, no matter how big or small.

What we focus on, we draw to ourselves. The universe wants to answer all of our hopes and prayers. But if we are focusing on the negative, we are not sending the right signals.

This is the law of attraction. Like attracts like. So, if we are focusing on the negative, it is no wonder negative situations will show up in our lives.

Think of it as reprogramming the brain. If you think of a negative… correct yourself and replace it with a positive. Say it 3 times out loud!

Whenever you encounter a situation, person, or instance in your life that you are grateful for, write it down on a slip of paper.

Set aside a jar, box or container. This is now your gratitude vessel. You can decorate it! Set it somewhere in your home where you will see it each day.

Whenever you write down a thing that you are grateful for, add it to your Gratitude Jar.

You can start this Gratitude Jar at any time of the year.

A nice practice is to open this Gratitude Jar on the 1st or the 2nd day of the new year. Read through all of the amazing things that have happened over the past year.

You can also randomly open the jar in times when you are lacking drive or feeling unmotivated. Sit in a quiet place with no distractions and read through your gratitude notes. Giving thanks and acknowledgement for all the amazing things that you have achieved. This really helps us to stay on our path. And also, to reinforce how far we have come.

Think of it as a goal list in reverse! There is nothing bad about writing a list of goals for the upcoming year(s). You may choose to do this in conjunction with your Gratitude Jar.

A Gratitude Jar is an easy way to stay in the present moment.

Gratitude Journals are also a lovely way to keep track of the amazing things happening in your life. There is no wrong or right way, but often putting something in writing really solidifies its existence and reinforces this in our soul and our brain.

Chapter 22
Meditation

"Inhale the future, Exhale the past."

Meditation is not as hard as it sounds. You don't need to sit for hours in silence to meditate.

It can be as simple as listening to a free YouTube meditation podcast, while sitting or lying comfortably on a chair or sofa.

Taking 10-15 minutes to meditate each day, can be truly life changing. Focus on what you would like to draw into your world, and what you would like to let go of.

Meditation can come in all different forms. From silent meditation, to chanting, to a candle meditation.

A teacher on one of my yoga teacher trainings taught us a beautiful and simple candlelight meditation. Light a candle. Dim the lights. Sitting comfortably in a chair or with crossed legs on a yoga mat, gaze at the candlelight. Focus, and let the thoughts of the world drift away. Choose an intention. It may be a promotion at work, a vacation you would like to take or even healing an issue in your life. Focus on this intention with no judgement or outcome attached. Focus on the breath. Long inhalations through the nose and long exhalations through the mouth.

Each time you become distracted or your focus shifts, slowly brings your focus back to the flame. Practice this for 5 minutes a few times a week. The outcome will surprise you.

Matras are another wonderful and powerful way to meditate. You can sing, chant or hum a Mantra. A Mantra is a simple phrase which is repeated. It brings the body and mind into alignment. It is hard to think other thoughts while singing a Mantra. It clears the mind and connects you to the divine.

Here are a few of my favorites:

- "Nam Myoho Renge Kyo" – Japanese Buddhist Mantra

- "Om Mani Padme Hum" – Nepalese Buddhist Mantra

- "I'm sorry, Please forgive me, Thank you, I love you." – The Ho'oponopono Hawaiian Mantra

- "Ohm" – The Universal sound of peace. This powerful Mantra can be repeated drawing focus to extending the sound. Inhale in and start the sound Ohm, exhaling the sound until it resonates in the chest and body

- "Ohm, Shanti, Shanti, Shanti" – Peace of mind, body and Speech, Indian Mantra

- ❖ "Om Vasudhare Svaha" – Attract abundance Mantra

Pranayama can be a form of meditation. Try a few of the breathing practices mentioned above. They can be especially helpful if you do not know where to begin with regards to adopting a meditation practice.

There is no right or wrong way to begin meditating. Try a few different methods and find out what works for you.

You can even start a meditation journal. Write down your thoughts, aspirations, and fears before you begin your practice and then again after you finish.

Notice any changes to your day when you meditate and when you do not.

THE SNEAKY AF* DIET BOOK

Chapter 23
How to Increase Neurotransmitters Naturally

NEUROTRANSMITTERS

ADRENALINE — fight or flight produced in stressful situations. Increases heart rate and blood flow, leading to physical boost and heightened awareness.	**GABA** — calming Calms firing nerves in the central nervous system. High levels improve focus, low levels cause anxiety. Also contributes to motor control and vision.
NORADRENALINE — concentration affects attention and responding actions in the brain. Contracts blood vessels, increasing blood flow.	**ACETYLCHOLINE** — learning Involved in thought, learning and memory. Activates muscle action in the body. Also associated with attention and awakening.
DOPAMINE — pleasure feelings of pleasure, also addiction, movement and motivation. People repeat behaviors that lead to dopamine release.	**GLUTAMATE** — memory Most common neurotransmitter. Involved in learning and memory, regulates development and creation of nerve contacts.
SEROTONIN — mood contributes to well-being and happiness. Helps sleep cycle and digestive system regulation. Affected by exercise and light exposure.	**ENDORPHINS** — euphoria Released during exercise, excitement and sex, producing well-being and euphoria, reducing pain

Neurotransmitter function is imperative in controlling our emotions, concentration, learning, gaining better sleep, libido and even pain perception. It is essential to have balanced neurotransmitters to live a happy, healthy life.

They can also affect a variety of feelings like joy, excitement, and happiness. Regulating these neurotransmitters can be easy by fueling our body with healthy, plant-based foods.

When we are deficient in one or more neurotransmitters, we can experience many issues such as sleeplessness, depression or lethargy. Our diet plays such an important role in the production and distribution of neurotransmitters. After all, we are what we eat!

Dopamine (excitatory)

Dopamine is an essential neurotransmitter that is created in the brain. We need a few things to survive. Water, food and dopamine! We also need air, human companionship and sleep… but most of all we need the above three.

So, what exactly is dopamine. Quite literally it is an essential chemical released by the brain when we experience something pleasurable. Examples of this can be, eating a nice meal, eating chocolate, drinking alcohol, savoring your morning cup of coffee or tea.

*'Dopamine is known as the **feel-good neurotransmitter**—a chemical that ferries information between neurons. The brain releases it when we eat foods that we crave, or while we have sex, contributing to feelings of pleasure and satisfaction as part of the reward system.' - Taken from healthdirect.com*

In the addicted brain, when a substance is consumed (for illustrative purposes we will use cocaine) dopamine levels are extremely elevated.

Normal dopamine levels are somewhere in the vicinity of **0 to 30 pg/mL – 80 pg/mL (195.8 pmol/L)**

These levels may increase to 100's of pg/ml when someone takes an addictive drug. This triggers the brain to 'crave' this experience, thus leading to a pattern of addiction.

In a depressed individual, or to a more extreme degree - a person with Parkinson's Disease, the dopamine levels are drastically reduced.

This can make it difficult for them to get out of bed, it can lead to decreased brain activity and trouble with motor skills.

Why am I pointing this out in a diet book? Because healthy dopamine levels are crucial to being healthy and happy.

I am also pointing this out, because as a person with quite severe ADHD, I have a personal relationship with needing to learn how to elevate my dopamine levels naturally. I always wondered why I was stuck in a loop of easily becoming addicted to/and craving specific substances and foods. It is because of a lack of dopamine in my brain!

ADHD is a gift. It helps me to complete tasks quickly. It can also mean I am trying to do several things at once.

I had to learn and research how to help myself. And the great news is that you too, can increase your dopamine levels naturally.

This will help you to feel happier and healthier. I promise!

Here is a short (but not complete list) of things you can do to elevate dopamine.

THE SNEAKY AF* DIET BOOK

- Meditation – yes Pranayama is included!

- Exercise

- Decreasing sugar intake

- Increasing protein consumption (yes beans, tofu and many vegan alternatives are included)

- Listening to Music! Yes, truly!

- Getting adequate sleep (6-8 hours per night)

- Maintaining a routine

- Decreasing Caffeine *(I know you probably don't want to hear this!)*

- Decreasing Alcohol Consumption *(I definitely don't want to hear this!)*

- Ensuring your diet includes adequate levels of Zinc, Vitamin C, Magnesium, Vitamin B6, Curcumin/Turmeric, Fish Oil, Vitamin D, Probiotics (Kombucha or Sauerkraut)

Without healthy levels of dopamine, we can feel depressed, unmotivated, and down.

Let's look at our last bullet point and expand of these a bit:

Zinc

Avocados! Delicious right? They are also very high in Zinc. Beans and nuts are not only a great source of protein – they are also high in Zinc.

Mushrooms and Kale are great plant-based ways to increase your zinc intake. They can be tasty and delicious too. (I have a great recipe for Portuguese Kale soup that is vegan and delicious)

Red meat and dairy can also be great sources of Zinc but if you are opting for a more plant-based diet, I want to illustrate that you needn't be afraid that you will miss out on specific important nutrients. They are all available on a plant-based diet. You just have to know what they are and make wise diet choices.

Vitamin C

If you feel you are not getting enough Vitamin C, I am an advocate of consuming a Liposomal C supplement that is derived from Sunflower Seeds.

There are many foods that can provide you with adequate Vitamin C though.

A few of these are: Citrus fruits (oranges, kiwi, lemon, grapefruit), Bell peppers (capsicum for those of you in Australia!), Strawberries, Tomatoes, Cruciferous vegetables (broccoli, Brussels sprouts, cabbage, cauliflower) and white potatoes.

Magnesium

Magnesium plays many crucial roles in the body, such as **supporting muscle and nerve function.** It is essential for the production of energy. It can also ensure better sleep patterns and a more restful night's rest. Low magnesium levels usually don't cause direct recognizable symptoms. However, chronically low levels can increase the risk of high blood pressure, heart disease, type 2 diabetes and even osteoporosis.

Here is a list of foods that will help ensure you are receiving enough Magnesium:

Pumpkin seeds, 30g (156mg), Chia seeds, 30 g (111mg), Almonds, 30g (80mg of magnesium), Spinach, boiled, ½ cup (78mg), Cashews, 30g (74mg), Peanuts, ¼ cup (63mg), soymilk, 1 cup (61mg)

Vitamin B6

Vitamin B-6 (pyridoxine) is important for normal brain development and for keeping the nervous system and immune system healthy.

I have always had a weird reaction to taking any kind of Vitamin B supplement. It can make me break out in hives! Fortunately, one of my favorite things in the world, Vegemite, is now available in Reduced Sodium with increased levels of Vitamins B6 & B12. And while I am not advocating that you go out and start eating vegemite, you could try it! You never know – you might even like it! It's a great addition to recipes for its beef-like flavor even though it is vegan.

Fortunately, there are foods that are naturally high in Vitamin B6:

Prunes, Apricots, Bananas, Plantains (Fried), Jackfruit which is a great meat alternative in tacos!

Curcumin/Turmeric

Turmeric is used extensively in recipes in India and Eastern countries. It has a distinct yellow color. Its most beneficial properties are curcuminoids.

Three of the best curcuminoids are curcumin, desmethoxycurcumin and bisdemethoxycurcumin.

Curcumin can lower inflammation in the body. Much of dis-ease (disease) in the west can be attributed to excessive inflammation in the body.

There are many curcumin supplements available on the market. Liquid curcumin is a great option as it is readily absorbable by the body.

Curcumin and Turmeric are also great anti-inflammatories and, as many doctors point out, inflammation in the body is the gateway to disease.

Vitamin D

The sun is a readily available source of vitamin D. Mushrooms are another great source of vitamin D and a great meat alternative.

Probiotics

More than 50% of dopamine is synthesized in the gut. Therefore, maintaining a healthy microbiome is super important. Probiotics can be extremely beneficial, as can eating foods that aid a healthy gut such as sauerkraut, and kimchi and drinking kombucha.

Most of the things we require we can get from our diet – providing it is a balanced and healthy diet. There's always margin for a bit of error, but I have personally found if I stick with my rule of 80/20 (80% plant based, 20% anything I like) then I can maintain a healthy weight easily, and I feel great! Really, I am probably at a 90% plant based and 10% animal products now.

Serotonin (inhibitory)

If dopamine is the pleasure neurotransmitter, then serotonin is the happiness neurotransmitter. Serotonin is produced in the gut, which is one extra reason to maintain a good healthy gut balance.

It is a chemical that carries messages to the brain and throughout the body.

Increasing serotonin naturally

- Exposure to bright sunlight. This is why we can feel down or lethargic in winter.

- Exercise. Even a 10 - 15 minute brisk walk can help increase serotonin.

- Diet! Read below for a list of foods that will naturally increase serotonin levels.

Pineapple

Pineapple contains high levels of bromelain which is a powerful anti-inflammatory. It also promotes healthy weight and digestion. Pineapple also contains tryptophan which helps to promote serotonin production.

Soy Products

Soy products have really gotten a bad rap over the past decade. They are actually really healthy and contain high levels of tryptophan. Freshly steamed soybeans (edamame) are a great source, as are tofu and soy milk.

Nuts & Seeds

If you can – opt for raw nuts and seeds and roast them yourself. This way you will cut down on the oil content. Cashews, pistachios, and almonds are all high in tryptophan which in turn promotes serotonin productivity in the intestines.

Dark Green Leafy Vegetables

Spinach, kale, asparagus, Brussels sprouts, Bok Choy, and avocados all help to increase serotonin levels.

Fermented Foods

Kimchi and sauerkraut are both excellent for good gut health and serotonin production. Yogurt is also good but always opt for full-fat fat unsweetened Greek yoghurt. You can always add granola and honey!

Norepinephrine – (excitatory)
(also known as Noradrenaline)

The parasympathetic nervous system is activated when you are not in danger. Things like deep breathing exercises, relaxing exercises, and even laughter can activate the parasympathetic nervous system. Listening to music or just plain relaxing also activates this.

On the flip side, you have the sympathetic nervous system which kicks in when you are in danger. When the body is in this mode for extended periods (fight or flight mode) many researchers believe it can increase your risk of diseases like obesity, cancer, and heart disease.

Norepinephrine is a chemical messenger and a neurotransmitter. It is responsible for releasing a stress hormone from the adrenal glands.

The amino acid tyrosine is necessary to produce norepinephrine, and tyrosine can also aid in weight loss. Tyrosine is produced by the body and is derived from the foods we consume.

Norepinephrine's main function is to protect the body from harm. Think of the olden days. You are out hunting for food (or gathering!) and a lion starts chasing you. Bingo! Norepinephrine kicks in.

You are in fight or flight mode.

You start to experience several sensations. You become more alert. Your focus is heightened. Your palms begin to sweat. Your pain tolerance becomes higher. Your reaction time becomes faster.

And hopefully, you run!

So why am I drawing attention to norepinephrine? Low levels of norepinephrine can cause many issues within the body.

- Depression

- Attention Deficit Disorder

- Fatigue

- Memory Loss

- Lack of Motivation

Here is a list of foods and things you can do that will help maintain healthy levels of norepinephrine:

Get More Exercise

A brisk 10-15 minute walk twice a day will help naturally elevate your levels of norepinephrine.

As will weight training, a bike ride, or any other form of exercise you choose to do!

Increase Quercetin intake

Quercetin not only increases levels of norepinephrine in the brain – it also helps elevate serotonin and dopamine.

Green tea is a wonderful natural source of quercetin. It may be time to think of switching out that morning cup o' joe with a nice cup of green tea instead.

Other foods that contain quercetin are apples and berries. Grapes also have high levels of quercetin. All the more reason to include fruit as a healthy snack.

As a side note, in the chapter on Trophology, the food combining chart suggests only eating fruit on its own.

It requires a specific environment for digestion. I am not suggesting giving up those delicious nut butter and banana sandwiches, whole grain pancakes and the like, but definitely consider eating this way (fruit + carbs) in moderation.

Melon is another interesting one as it requires its own specific digestive environment and should only be eaten alone.

Foods that naturally balance norepinephrine

- Almonds

- Avocado

- Bananas

- Lima Beans

- Pumpkin Seeds

- Sesame Seeds

Glutamate (excitatory)

Glutamate is an essential neurotransmitter for your brain. It plays an important role in memory and learning. It helps to regulate mood and is important for maintaining a healthy sleeping cycle.

Low levels of glutamate can cause depression, trouble concentrating, lack of sleep, low energy levels and exhaustion.

Glutamate and GABA are the most plentiful neurotransmitters in the human body, with GABA making up about 1/3 of all neurotransmitters. They are opposites – Glutamate being excitatory and GABA being inhibitory.

A balance between these neurotransmitters is crucial. They have a homeostatic relationship and work to keep each other in balance.

High levels can also have negative impacts on your health and may lead to diseases such as Parkinsons Disease.

You can naturally regulate glutamate by:

- Consuming foods rick in Omega 3's
- Meditation & Relaxation
- Increase vitamin C intake
- Increase magnesium intake

- Increase Vitamin D intake – sunshine is your best source of vitamin D. A walk in the sun daily for 15-20 minutes can provide you with Vitamin D.

Omega 3 rich foods

Flax seeds, chia seeds and walnuts are all high in Omega 3's. Soybeans are also high in Omega 3's and are super delicious. I like to buy the whole soybeans (in the shell) frozen and I steam them for 6-8 minutes. You can add sea salt, everything but the bagel or a spicy sauce to add flavor.

Oily fish are also a wonderful source of Omega 3's. Salmon, mackerel, sardines and anchovies are great in small amounts. I always choose wild caught and not farm raised.

Vitamin C

Citrus fruits are a great source of vitamin C. Kiwi fruits, oranges and grapefruit are best eaten whole (not juiced) as they contain essential vital fiber.

Strawberries and tomatoes are also high in Vitamin C.

Delicious green leafy vegetables such as cabbage, cauliflower, broccoli and Brussel sprouts are good sources.

Vitamin D

Sunshine is your best source of vitamin D. A walk in the sun daily for 15-20 minutes can provide you with enough Vitamin D. Don't forget your sunscreen! I like to walk/exercise before 10am or after 4pm.

Magnesium

Here is a list of foods that will help ensure you are receiving enough Magnesium:

Pumpkin seeds, 30g (156mg), Chia seeds, 30 g (111mg), Almonds, 30g (80mg of magnesium), Spinach, boiled, ½ cup (78mg), Cashews, 30g (74mg), Peanuts, ¼ cup (63mg), soymilk, 1 cup (61mg)

GABA (inhibitory)

GABA and Glutamate and important neurotransmitters. There are many things to make our neurotransmitters get out of whack. Understanding foods and ways to increase production of neurotransmitters is key to wellness and good health.

GABA is essential to our fight and flight mechanism. It is associated with a sense of calm and reducing anxiety. Think of it as a natural Xanax! Glutamate is the opposite. It is responsible for a feeling of excitement. Glutamate is essential as it breaks down into GABA; without adequate Glutamate levels we cannot make GABA.

GABA supports gut motility, and it also reduces inflammation. It is created in the brain.

Glutamate is synthesized by Glutamine. Eating too much protein can inhibit our production of Glutamate and in turn our production of GABA.

Low levels of GABA can result in depression!

THE SNEAKY AF* DIET BOOK

The great news is – you do not have to go out and buy a bunch of supplements. There are many natural ways to increase your GABA levels.

Foods that increase GABA naturally:

- Foods Containing Soy
- Fermented foods like Sauerkraut and Kim Chi
- Citrus Fruits – oranges, mandarins, lemons, blood oranges
- Walnuts and Almonds
- Sweet Potatoes
- Green leafy vegetables like Spinach and Broccoli
- Dark cocoa – yes dark chocolate! Yum!
- Berries – raspberries, blueberries, black currants, blackberries
- Brown Rice
- Lentils (a great replacement for ground beef)
- Green Tea
- Shrimp and Halibut (in moderation)

Exercise! Yoga and meditation have been shown to increase GABA levels.

Avoid excessive alcohol and junk food – these have all a negative impact on GABA levels. Adding essential oils to a diffuser can help increase GABA levels: Lavender, Bergamot, Lemon balm, Valerian, Jasmine, Chamomile.

Essential oils can be added to a diffuser next to your bed. They can help you sleep better and increase neurotransmitters while you are sleeping.

This is a wonderful way to combat insomnia!

Acetylcholine (excitatory)

Acetylcholine is a neurotransmitter that plays an important role in learning, memory, arousal, and involuntary muscle movement.

It has many important functions within the body.

It aids in digestion by moving food through the intestines. It contracts intestinal muscles (involuntarily), and aids in secreting digestive juices.

It regulates heart contractions and regulates the flow of blood throughout the body.

It causes glands to secrete tears, sweat and saliva (not just digestive juices!).

It regulates the adrenal glands and signals them to release of adrenaline and norepinephrine.

It controls the release and flow of urine. And in men, it causes an erection.

Foods that helps regulate Acetylcholine:

- Nuts including almonds, peanuts and pistachios
- Kidney beans
- Green beans
- Mung beans
- Peas
- Soy products such as tofu and soy milk
- Green vegetables
- Eggplant
- Fruits including figs, oranges, and strawberries

Meditation, pranayama, and yoga can all increase acetylcholine naturally. Antihistamines can decrease levels and should be avoided unless necessary.

Chapter 24
Enduro India -
The Adventure of a Lifetime

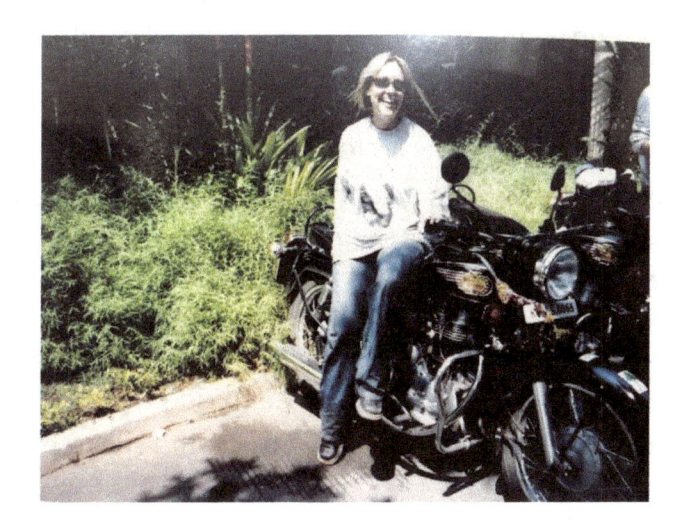

Why am I including this chapter – because apparently, I am an adrenaline or possibly more to the point a dopamine junkie.

So, I was in a bar in England with my English husband (ex-husband now). We had probably been drinking a few too many pints.

One of my best friends in America, whom I will refer to as CW, in the hopes of keeping his anonymity, had recently bought a rather expensive house in Corona Del Mar.

As I had shown him property in the past (being a realtor for 7 years in California before I moved to England) I insisted his realtor pay me a referral fee.

I was most excited to receive my rather handsome check and what did I do? Went straight to the Harley Davidson dealership in London and bought myself a spanking brand new 2003 anniversary edition sportster motorcycle.

I had grown up riding motorcycles. My friends and I used to swap our ponies in exchange for a zoom around on a dirt bike with the local guys who lived in our neighborhood. The guys probably liked us. We didn't care.

We grew up near a creek with riding paths for hundreds of miles. Back then, in the 80's people were free to ride their motorcycles, horses, bicycles etc on these paths. So, I could ride a motorbike. Not well but I could ride.

In America, I decided to pass my motorcycle test. We rented a sportster for the day, and I really wasn't the greatest road rider. Maybe I was a bit rusty.

When I told my friend CW that I had spent the referral commission check on a new Harley Davidson he exclaimed that he never would have agreed to this if he knew this was how I was going to spend the money!

Anyway, back to the story. We were drinking in this pub and there was a wall of postcards advertising different holidays and vacation things to do and see. There was one that stood out.

Ten whole days riding around India on a Royal Enfield motorcycle! And it was for a great cause. All of the participants were required to raise at least three-thousand pounds sterling (about $5,500 USD) for the cause. The Royal Enfields would then be donated to park rangers at the completion of the ride. The extra money would go towards building a hospital for Pain and Palliative Care in southern India.

This was it! The English husband and I shook on it! We were going back to India. It was one of the places we had been lucky enough to visit several times previously and we absolutely loved it.

I think this was around September of 2003. As you may well know, England gets increasing cold and rainy during the winter months. My plan had been to put a couple of thousand miles on the Harley Sportster in preparation.

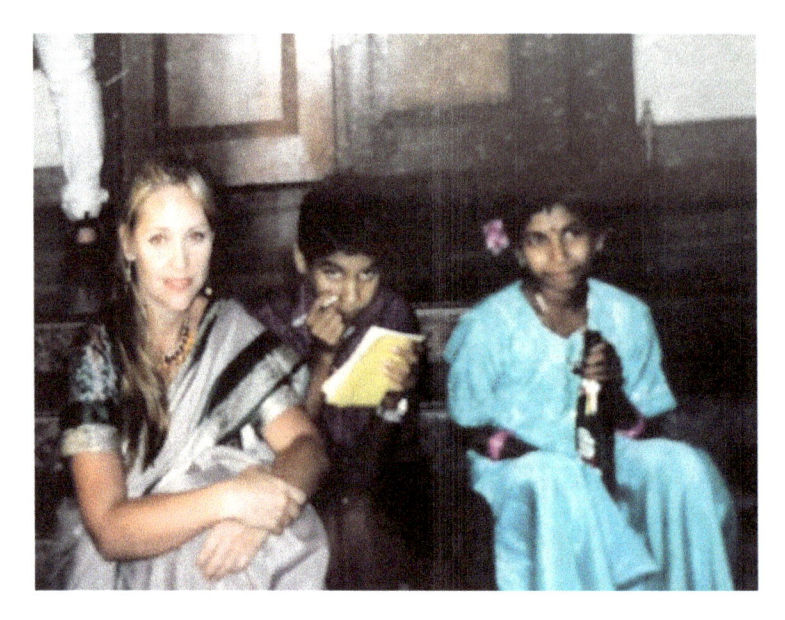

What actually happened was I rode around 100 miles. The Enduro India trip was in March. I was studying photography full-time in London so the idea of becoming a better rider was put on the back burner.

I vividly remember assembling with 80 other riders at London Heathrow. We were ready to go to India.

Well, they were but I probably wasn't ready to ride a motorcycle for 8 – 10 hours a day.

I survived it! I did it. I was frightened and nervous every day. But it was truly one of the greatest trips and experiences of my life.

How does this fit in with the Sneaky Diet Book? The people of Kerala and Tamil Nadu in India are primarily vegetarian folk. The food was amazing.

Despite the fact that some days I had to eat with my dirty motorcycle-riding hands (no knives or forks at the lunch restaurants). The other interesting fact is that they rarely consume alcohol.

In fact, the team that organized the ride would have to call ahead to the hotels to tell them… 'No, we need more beer!' In fact, cases and cases of beer. We often ran out of beer around 9 or 10 pm at night which was probably a good thing as we were up at 5 am to have breakfast and start riding again!

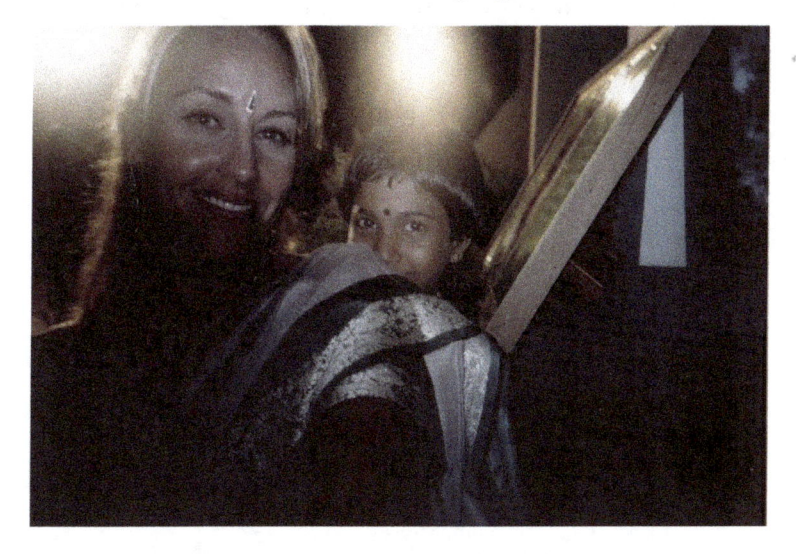

I believe we collectively raised over 200,000 GBP (British Pounds Sterling). We helped to build a hospital. We helped house and pay tuition for two HIV positive children who had been ostracized by their community and were not allowed to go to school. Their parents had both passed away. We hired a private tutor and paid for their accommodation in advance for the next 10 years.

Eating this way not only made me feel great, but I believe it helped me meet the challenge of the immense focus and concentration that was required to complete this exhausting but rewarding motorcycle ride.

Unfortunately, when I returned to England this adoption of eating healthily did not stick.

I returned to eating according to the laws of Trophology (food combining). I would eat primarily carbs in the morning, fruits and vegetables from 10 am-4 pm, and meat and green vegetables at night.

When you look at this diet – it really is 2/3rd vegan. It is not a bad alternative if you are on the fence about giving up meat, but you'd like to lose weight.

Chapter 25
A Plant-based Week

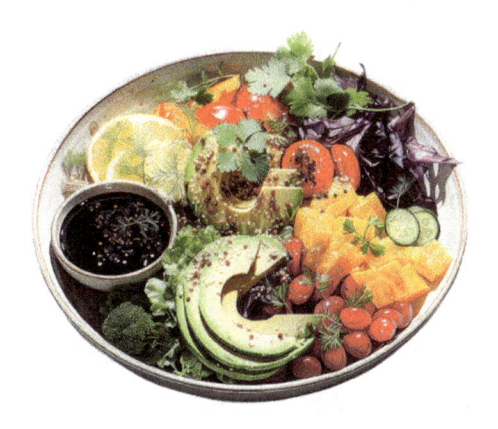

This is a basic meal planner. I have not included the full recipes because they are plentiful online. Just type in the word 'vegan' after each recipe and you will have loads of options.

Hopefully, you have already started adding some vegan meals to your days. Or, if you are on the fence as to where or how to start – choose one day a week where you will eat entirely plant-based. I like this option as it gives your body a 24-hour break from meat and dairy.

Plan out what you are going to eat. Make a list of ingredients you might need. Go shopping and make sure you have extra snacks and healthy options in case you are hungry between meals. Nuts are a great way to go as they are filling and healthy.

Once you factor in a day, take note of how you feel and how you sleep on that particular day. Then add another day. And another. Before you know it you be eating plant-based 50% of the time. And then 60%... 70%... 80%. It's that easy!

Take note of how your clothes fit after a few weeks. Does your skin look clearer? Is your mind clearer? I find eating plant-based not only gives me more energy, but it also helps me to focus and think more clearly.

If you do feel better, add another day or two a week. By this time, you will have some delicious plant-based recipes down. You will notice your taste buds are changing.

On the flip side, if you don't feel better, analyze the foods you chose – add more fruits and vegetables. In winter, add more soups with vegetables and stir-fries.

You are doing great! **Now, keep it going!**

MONDAY	BREAKFAST	Oatmeal with almond milk, cinnamon, maple syrup, nut butter, banana/fruit, raisins
	LUNCH	Tomato, olive, and hummus bagel. Side of couscous or quinoa
	DINNER	Veggie fajitas with black beans, red pepper, purple onion, and mushrooms with veggie tortillas and vegan cheese
	SNACKS	Almonds, banana, orange, sunflower seeds

THE SNEAKY AF* DIET BOOK

TUESDAY	BREAKFAST	Spiced lentils on whole grain toast with vegan butter alternative. Try wholegrain or fully sprouted toast!
	LUNCH	Deviled potato sandwich with celery and mustard. Add arugula or make it into a side salad
	DINNER	Buddha bowl with roasted sweet potato, kale, chickpeas, veggies and tahini dressing
	SNACKS	Popcorn, hummus and celery or crackers, oreo cookies, fruit

WEDNESDAY	BREAKFAST	Breakfast wrap with tortilla, soyrizo,/vegan meat alternative, hash browns, onions and peppers, and 1 egg/egg alternative
	LUNCH	Roasted cauliflower salad with couscous and roasted vegetables
	DINNER	Falafel sandwich will quick pickle red onions, spinach, tomato and cucumber
	SNACKS	Home roasted cashews with maple syrup and everything but the bagel seasoning

THURSDAY	BREAKFAST	Chia seed pudding (made the night before) with almond milk, vanilla essence, honey or maple syrup, banana, and strawberries
	LUNCH	Citrus lime tofu salad with butter lettuce and a spicy chili dressing. Add roasted peanuts for crunch
	DINNER	Sarah's Carbonara. If you can't find benevolent bacon, mushrooms work great too!
	SNACKS	Avocado and crackers with tajin, dry roasted almonds, fruit smoothie with almond milk

FRIDAY	BREAKFAST	Nut butter and banana on toast with an almond milk and fruit smoothie
	LUNCH	Coconut curry with vegetables, mushrooms and rice, add some roasted cashews
	DINNER	Indian korma curry with spiced lentils and naan bread or sub rice for the bread
	SNACKS	Vegan cookies (you deserve it), vegan chocolate energy balls with maca, pecans

SATURDAY	BREAKFAST	Apple and oatmeal pancakes with maple syrup and walnuts. Make a few extra and save them in the fridge as a snack
	LUNCH	Left over coconut curry from last night. Can be served cold over salad
	DINNER	Soba noodles with miso and vegetables. Add mushrooms and tofu to add protein
	SNACKS	Siete Vegan Ranch chips with guacamole and salsa, a cup of skinny pop (popcorn), dried figs

SUNDAY	BREAKFAST	Roasted Sweet potato and lentil quesadillas with vegan cheese sauce
	LUNCH	Acai bowl with blueberries, banana, goji berries and nut butter
	DINNER	Vegan superfood grain bowl with edamame, avocado, beet and roasted peanuts
	SNACKS	Nut butter stuffed dates, pistachios, cup of berries, energy bite (homemade)

Chapter 26
Be Part of the Plant-based Revolution!

Congratulations on your decision to help change this beautiful planet we are all lucky enough to live on! The change starts with you.

Just by deciding to make the simple step to shift a few meals each day, or each week to eating plants can change your health for the better and it can help save the environment too!

Its fact-based. Many doctors and nutritionists are jumping on board and spreading the word that you can be every bit as healthy and strong, by eating plant-based rather than eating *dead things*.

Now, there are so many alternatives in grocery stores and restaurants. And the great news is that the more demand for these products, the more companies will have to pivot and provide more alternatives at a competitive price.

Be part of the change. Say no to GMOs. Say no to the pointless slaughter of animals.

Say yes to losing weight!

Say yes to eating delicious healthy food!

Say yes to having more energy and feeling healthier.

Now pat yourself on the back for committing to making the single most important dietary change you can possibly make.

And prepare to not only look amazing but to feel amazing too!

Chapter 26
Can I Eat Plant-Based Entirely and Be Healthy?

Absolutely! In fact, many athletes and Olympians eat entirely vegan diets. Eating an entirely plant-based diet will decrease your risk of heart disease, cancer, high cholesterol and reduce inflammation in the body.

There are a few considerations though. Eating entirely plant-based can make it hard to receive the amount of Vitamin B12 your body requires. Fortunately, nutritional yeast (our wonderful cheese alternative) is high in Vitamin B12.

Avocados and mushrooms are also wonderful clean sources of B12. Avocados are a wonderful addition to smoothies. Their creaminess makes them a great alternative to sour cream. They contain a healthy unsaturated form of fat and they can help to lower cholesterol.

Fish like salmon and mackerels are great sources of Vitamin B12 and eaten a few times a week they can help to maintain healthy levels of Omega 3 fatty acids and vitamins. You can receive enough Omega 3 fatty acids by ensuring you add flax seeds, chia seeds, walnuts, soybeans, and hemp seeds to your diet. Seeds can be sprinkled onto salads, soups, and sandwiches to add a wonderful texture and flavor.

Calcium is another concern when eating vegan. Provided you eat lots of beans, peas, lentils, and nuts such as almonds and hazelnuts you will receive enough calcium. Tahini paste is a wonderful additive to salad dressing, sauces, and recipes and it is high in calcium.

Seaweed and dark leafy greens are also wonderful clean sources of calcium. Many people complain of gassiness when consuming large amounts of beans. Adding a small sheet of seaweed to your beans, chickpeas, or lentils will prevent this! Just add the sheet of seaweed to your pot of beans while you are cooking them and it will add a pleasant saltiness and prevent a rumbling tummy!

Vitamin D is necessary to absorb calcium. Our best source of Vitamin D is sunshine! 10-15 minutes in the sun each day will provide you with enough vitamin D although this can be difficult in colder climates. Shitake mushrooms are a wonderful source of Vitamin D.

Many of the nut milk alternatives are now fortified with Vitamin D and calcium. And whilst it is always better to receive Vitamins and minerals from your diet, sometimes supplements are necessary.

Protein and Iron are considerations to take note of when eating entirely vegan. Provided you are eating a variety of nuts, seeds, whole grains, lentils, beans, and green leafy vegetables you will find it easy to maintain your iron and protein levels. Nut butter is a wonderful addition to smoothies, desserts, and sauces.

Selenium is a mineral found in soil. While we only require a small amount of selenium it is essential for metabolism.

Fortunately, you can receive adequate levels of selenium by eating asparagus, brazil nuts, mushrooms, sesame seeds, sunflower seeds, tofu, and whole grains.

Who Should Not Eat Vegan?

I would personally say children and adolescents should not eat entirely plant-based as they require many calories and a variety of foods to fuel their growing bodies. There have only been limited studies conducted on vegan vs omnivore children and the main concern is a lack of adequate calcium in the vegan diet.

Another concern would be women adopting a fully vegan diet whilst pregnant or breastfeeding. While they could eat a completely balanced diet primarily made up of plant based foods, it would be advisable to supplement their diet with healthy lean meats and some dairy products.

Chapter 27
Be Part of the Plant-based Revolution!

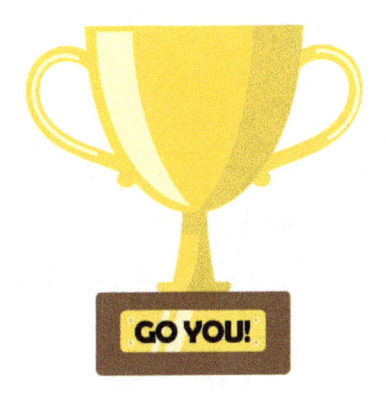

Congratulations on your decision to help change this beautiful planet we are all lucky enough to live on! The change starts with you.

Just by deciding to make the simple step to shift a few meals each day, or each week to eating plants can change your health for the better and it can help save the environment too!

Its fact-based. Many doctors and nutritionists are jumping on board and spreading the word that you can be every bit as healthy and strong, by eating plant-based rather than eating *dead things*.

Now, there are so many alternatives in grocery stores and restaurants. And the great news is that the more demand for these products, the more companies will have to pivot and provide more alternatives at a competitive price.

Be part of the change. Say no to GMOs. Say no to the pointless slaughter of animals.

Say yes to losing weight!

Say yes to eating delicious healthy food!

Say yes to having more energy and feeling healthier.

Now pat yourself on the back for committing to making the single most important dietary change you can make.

And prepare to not only look amazing but to feel amazing too!

Glossary of Plant Medicines

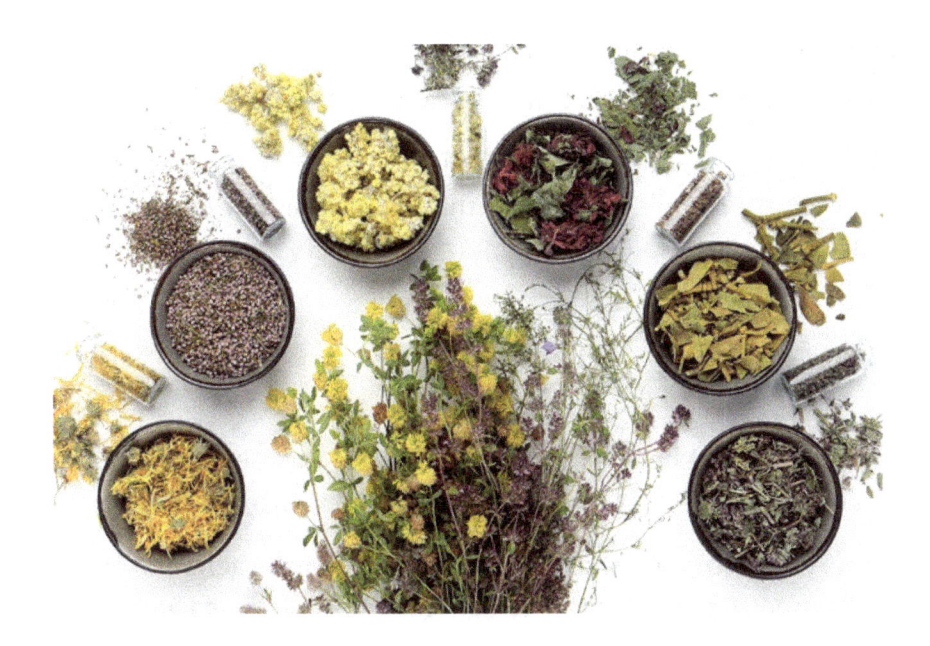

Plant medicine can be an effective alternative to traditional Western medicine. I am not advocating that you choose plant medicine as a preference over pharmaceutical drugs if you have an illness or life-threatening condition.

It serves an important function if you have an issue that can easily be resolved without taking pharmaceuticals. The main issue in Western medicine is that we are taught to merely mask the symptoms of many ailments without getting to the root cause.

This is where plant medicine comes into the equation. Often it can be used to treat issues such as inflammation, pain, anxiety, indigestion, lack of sleep, headaches, fatigue, stress etc. It can effectively do this by getting to the root cause and alleviating the ailment. This is far preferable to just getting rid of the symptoms without truly curing the cause. Often pharmaceuticals can present a whole new set of symptoms without even curing the ailment you are treating! Then you will need to take another medication to mask those symptoms, which in turn may cause more side effects.

I will outline a few of the popular plant medicines that can be used, and most are completely legal in the USA at the time of writing this book.

Aloe Vera

It is an incredibly healing plant. It is effective for calming sunburn to expedite the healing of a wound. Aloe reduces inflammation.

It is very easy to grow, and it is a handy plant to have at home. The sap can be used as part of a facial to tighten pores. It has also been shown to calm acne and skin rashes.

It can be ingested to help with digestive issues. I strongly recommend purchasing aloe specifically for internal use. It can calm indigestion, relieve constipation, and treat ulcerative colitis.

Ashwagandha

Ashwagandha is most commonly used as an anti-anxiety plant medicine. It can help with insomnia too.

It is also used for memory and mental clarity.

Several clinical trials have been conducted on Ashwagandha. It has proved effective in reducing cortisol within the body and alleviating stress and anxiety.

Ashwagandha may also prove effective for reducing blood sugar levels which could prove to be advantageous for anyone pre-diabetic.

Calendula

Calendula has wonderful orange flowers. It can attract butterflies and it's a pretty house plant. It's easy to grow in a plant pot in full sun.

Calendula is great for treating dermatitis, eczema, and rashes. It has anti-inflammatory properties.

It can be used by drying the flowers and infusing them in tea. Calendula oil is also common, and it is often added to skincare products.

Cannabidiol

Cannabidiol (CBD) is a plant medicine I have become very familiar with over the past 5 years. It is a non-psychoactive cannabinoid derived from the hemp plant containing less than 0.3% THC. This means it does not have the 'high' associated with cannabis.

I helped run a successful CBD company with a retail store and online business in Southern California for 5 years.

Having witnessed firsthand the profound benefits of treating our customers/patients with CBD I am a huge advocate of its healing powers. I have witnessed its incredible benefits in treating many of the above-mentioned ailments.

And while it does not work effectively for every individual, it is a worthwhile plant medicine to seek out and try. If you suffer from pain and inflammation.

We all have an Endocannabinoid System (ECS) which is made up of 3 parts:

- A widespread network of cannabinoid receptors (CB1 & CB2)
- Endogenous cannabinoids (endocannabinoids) such as AEA & 2-AG
- Endocannabinoid metabolic enzymes such as FAAH and MAGL3

When we are deficient in specific endocannabinoids we can experience increased pain, inflammation, and an array of other symptoms. Research studies have shown that sufferers of PTSD are often deficient in 2-AG suggesting the body's inability to reset e-CB and restore homeostasis.

The ECS is responsible for homeostasis within the body. It helps to regulate:

- Immune Function
- Memory and Learning
- Temperature control
- Cardiovascular System
- Sleep
- Pain Control
- Emotional Processing
- Inflammatory Response

Fortunately, the cannabinoids derived from the plant *cannabis sativa* (CBD) can be used in place of the endocannabinoids the body would usually make. These cannabinoids can be derived from a plant high in THC or from the hemp plant which is naturally low in THC (the psychoactive component in marijuana) and high in CBD which is not psychoactive.

There are over 113 Phyto cannabinoids that scientists have discovered in CBD. Its lack of psychoactive effects and low instances of side effects make it an ideal treatment for pain, inflammation, insomnia, anxiety, and depression.

CBD is just one of a plethora of plant-based medicinal alternatives to treat an array of ailments. CBD is not a cure for many ongoing illnesses like arthritis, but it can help to manage symptoms effectively and naturally with little to no side effects.

Chamomile

Chamomile is often used to combat anxiety and stress. Chamomile-infused teas are a wonderful nighttime beverage to help ensure a restful night's sleep.

It is often used to reduce inflammation and swelling. A poultice can be made to apply to a strain or injury.

The tea can be used to relieve nausea and vomiting.

Curcumin

Curcumin is a wonderful anti-inflammatory. It has been used widely to prevent the pain caused by arthritis. Curcumin is an active ingredient of the spice turmeric, which has been used in Indian cooking for thousands of years.

Curcumin may aid in killing cancer cells. It could also be cancer-preventative. Curcumin has been reported to modulate cancer growth factors.

Curcumin contains a polyphenol that has been shown to target multiple signaling molecules at the cellular level. It has shown very promising in reducing cancerous tumors in lab tests on animals, although human trials have not been conclusive enough due to limited data.

Echinacea

The leaf stalk and root of the Echinacea plant is most commonly used to shorten the length of a cold or upper respiratory infection.

It is often found in tablet form and is regularly combined with Goldenseal. It is high in antioxidants as it contains compounds called alkamides.

Echinacea may help to lower blood sugar levels by restricting the amount of sugar entering the blood. Not enough research has been done on this, however, and Echinacea is not recommended for long-term use.

Milk Thistle Extract

Milk Thistle extract is available in capsule form at most health food stores and online retailers. It is an amazing, healing herb.

It can help to protect your liver. It has been used for centuries to treat gallbladder and liver issues. It may help regenerate liver tissue.

Milk thistle has anti-inflammatory and antioxidant properties. Preliminary studies have shown milk thistle to reduce plaque in the brain which is the precursor to Alzheimer's Disease.

Its neuroprotective qualities could help prevent oxidization in the brain.

I take milk thistle each morning as a preventative measure. It is definitely worth taking if you enjoy the odd glass of wine.

Saw Palmetto

Saw Palmetto is a palm tree found in Africa and The Caribbean. It was used by The Seminole Tribe to help boost fertility.

It has been used to reduce enlarged prostate and it has proved effective for treating urinary tract infections.

It has been shown effective for aiding in relieving the need to urinate frequently during the night.

Tea Tree Oil

Tea tree oil originates from Australia. Melaleuca oil is an oil derived from the tea tree plant.

It is generally safe to use topically although it can be toxic when ingested. The oil is not recommended to be used in a diffuser around animals.

It is effective in treating acne, athletes' foot, dandruff, lice, and nail fungus. It is anti-inflammatory.

It can help to benefit the respiratory system and help to heal upper respiratory infections when added to a diffuser.

These last two are not currently legal in the USA.

Psilocybin (Magic Mushrooms)

Magic Mushrooms have been used by indigenous leaders for centuries. They have long believed in the power of the female spirit of the mushroom to heal illness and disease.

Indian tribal leaders have long used Peyote in ceremonial gatherings to summon the spirit of Mother Earth to resolve conflict, create community, and heal.

In fact, the use of psychedelics dates back to the Roman Era when a chalice was discovered to contain traces of a mind-altering substance that was believed to have been given to the smartest and brightest to help them foresee events and learn from the universe.

I am not advocating that you go out and buy illegal magic mushrooms from a guy with dreadlocks on a street corner. I am saying, however, that these types of drugs have a time and a place. It is in a clinical setting, under a doctor's supervision. This usually only happens when all other avenues of treatment have been exhausted and have been rendered unsuccessful.

There is an amazing foundation in Northern California called MAPS. They have been studying the effects of many plant medicines that have previously been classified as drugs and placed on a banned schedule list making them illegal.

MAPS has done amazing clinical trials which have shown that many of these illicit substances have far greater potential for treating PTSD, trauma, and illness than their pharmaceutical alternatives.

We are nearing an age where magic mushrooms will soon become legal in many States in the USA.

DMT (Ayahuasca)

At the time of writing this Ayahuasca is not legal in the USA. It is definitely not recommended for anyone with pre-existing medical conditions or people taking medications prescribed by a doctor. It can be dangerous.

I have been fortunate enough to take part in several Ayahuasca ceremonies. While I do not recommend that it is something you would do recreationally, it has a purpose in helping people to heal.

I watched an interview with Prince Harry and Anderson Cooper recently where Prince Harry talked about taking ayahuasca to deal with the emotional trauma of losing his mother. I completely get it. Ayahuasca helped me to deal with trauma.

It's an extreme measure. But I don't ever do things by halves.

And here's what I will tell you. It changed my life. It gave me a purpose. I would not be writing this book or working in the field of plant medicine if I had not gone to that first plant medicine retreat in Peru.

So probably don't do it unless you are ready and willing for your life to change.

THE SNEAKY AF* DIET BOOK

A fellow yogi once told me the story of her friend who was a stockbroker in Sydney, Australia. Great life. Making oodles and oodles of money.

Did ayahuasca.

Quit his job.

He then moved to the outback in Australia and became a wilderness guide showing tourists around Uluru (formerly Ayers Rock).

Your life can profoundly change by taking plant medicines. And the food you eat is medicine!

Acknowledgements

For my Mum – I love you more than anyone on the planet. Thank you for being there for me through all of my trials and tribulations, and for understanding, and loving me unconditionally.

To Dr Clifford Corman – without the diagnosis of ADHD at age 45 years of age, this book would not have been possible.

To the CBD and Plant Medicine industry – thank you to this community for sharing your wealth of information and healing.

To Mother Earth (Gaia/Aya) – I hope we can do better. Collectively, I know we can!

Great Resources

Books

The China Study: The Most Comprehensive Study of Nutrition Ever Conducted and the Startling Implications for Diet, Weight Loss, and Long-term Health
by T. Colin Campbell

Forks Over Knives—The Cookbook: Over 300 Simple and Delicious Plant-Based Recipes to Help You Lose Weight, Be Healthier, and Feel Better Every Day
by Del Sroufe

How Not to Die: Discover the Foods Scientifically Proven to Prevent and Reverse Disease
by Michael Grege

The Complete Guide to Vegan Food Substitutions: Veganize It! Foolproof Methods for Transforming Any Dish into a Delicious New Vegan Favorite
by Celine Steen

Veganomicon: The Ultimate Vegan Cookbook
by Isa Chandra Moskowitz

Vodka is Vegan – A Manifesto for Living Better and Not Being An Asshole
by Matt & Phil Letten

Podcasts

- The Rich Roll Podcast

- The Plant-based Morning Show

- The Exam Room Podcast

- The Plant-Powered People Podcast

Movies

The Game Changers (2019)

What The Health (2017)

The Animal People (2019)

Cowspiracy – The Sustainability Secret (2014)

Fed Up (2014)

Seaspiracy (2021

Printed in the USA
CPSIA information can be obtained
at www.ICGtesting.com
LVHW022343030524
779162LV00002B/377